"Coach JC's Gameplan delivers the truth about how the mind is an incredibly powerful weapon. It shows you how mastering your mindset can be the tool to obtaining anything that you want in life. The power of my mind has been the engine that has driven me through all life's obstacles, both on and off the court. The Secret To Real Weight Loss Success is the coaching that will change your life forever."

Samuel Dalembert
NBA-Pro Basketball Player

"Coach JC's 27 day game plan will transform your life. As business owners and moms, we definitely have more energy for our busy careers and families. If you want success, The Secret To Real Weight Loss Success is a must!"

Deedra Determan and Melanie Henry
Co-Founders, 918moms.com

"Having been in the fitness industry since 1985 and the chiropractic profession since 1995, I have seen a lot of programs come and go! What comes and stays are proven-effective principles and the power to apply them. This book will provide you with both! While reading this book I could hear Coach JC's voice coaching me...just like he does in person. Whether you are coaching with him through The Secret To Real Weight Loss Success or live, the results are the same...exactly what your mind determines to achieve. He will help you do just that...one way or another!"

Dr. Shannon
Coach JC's Chiropractor, Inspirational Speaker, Author
Founder of health4life REVOLUTiON!
www.cornerstone4life.com

"Through simple 8-step workouts and self-reflective mental exercises, Jonathan Conneely takes you through a revitalizing 27-day journey with The Secret To Real Weight Loss Success program. Anyone who is looking to truly change and transform--from the inside out--needs to pick up this book."

Joel Marion, CISSN, NSCA-CPT
Author of The Cheat to Lose Diet

"Coach JC has a passion to help those achieve true success in their lives that extends far beyond just their physical well-being. With his physical fitness system he has found a way to reinvigorate people of all ages to achieve their dreams physically, mentally and financially. His book is a must read for anyone who is serious about achieving life balance and true success."

Clay Clark
USA Small Business Administration Entrepreneur of the Year
www.MakeYourLifeEpic.com

The Secret to Real Weight Loss Success

ISBN: 978-0-88144-510-7

Copyright © 2010 by Jonathan Conneely

Published by

Total Publishing and Media

9731 East 54th Street

Tulsa, OK 74146

www.totalpublishingandmedia.com

THE SECRET TO *real* WEIGHT LOSS SUCCESS

Your 27 Day
Body Transformation Gameplan

THE SECRET TO REAL WEIGHT LOSS SUCCESS
COACH JC'S MISSION

My mission for The Secret To Real Weight Loss Success is for it to help over one million people to not only lose weight and get into the best shape of their lives, but to take control of their lives for good! My goal is that this book will be the turning point in the reader's life so that he or she can live his or her greatest life and fulfill his or her destiny.

THE SECRET TO REAL WEIGHT LOSS SUCCESS
YOUR 27 DAY BODY TRANSFORMATION GAMEPLAN!

ACKNOWLEDGEMENTS

First, I want to thank God for giving me the burning passion to help people succeed and live their lives to the fullest. For the wisdom, insight, and clarity on how to get my message across to the people. For the compassion and sensitivity that He has given me for other human beings and the passion that burns so strongly inside of me to see others live their lives to the fullest.

To my mother, who has made me the person I am today and has supported me in every dream and goal that I have ever had. Her will to win and to never give up has motivated me to be better in all that I do. To my sister, Jaime, my best friend, who has made me a better person and has motivated me with her confidence and assertiveness in life. Mom, Jaime – I love you both so much and thank you for always being there AND FOR HELPING ME through the tough times. I can honestly say that without the both of you, I would not be the man that I am to-day and possibly would not even be here today. You are my role models and I am indebted to you both for life!

To my lovely fiancée, Jodi: thank you for all your support and standing by my side throughout the years, I am grateful and blessed to have such a special woman by my side, and I wouldn't trade you for anything! I look forward to spending my future with you. To my daughter, Alivia: I love you very much and you motivate me on a daily basis to be my best. Everything that I do I do it for you! I love you and I will always be the best father I can be for you.

To my father: thanks for always being you and thank you for all of your support and love over the years. To all of my family and friends – too many of you to name – but you know who you are. I love you and appreciate all the support.

To my buddy, employee, partner, and friend, Nate: thank you for all of your hard work and dedication. Thank you for buying into my vision and helping it to become a reality. Go and play a round of golf now, bro!

To everyone who has helped me through the years to make this book a reality: all the knowledge that you have imparted into me and all your support and motivation is why this book has been completed. Pastor Billy Joe Daugherty, thank you for all of the inspiration, knowledge and wisdom that you have imparted into me! Sammy D, "The Haitian Sicilian," Jack, "Fake it til you make it!" To the whole ORU family! To Cheyenne, my little friend and helper, I love you and you are a SURVIVOR!

To the entire Bootcamp Tulsa Family, I love you all and let's keep living life to the fullest.

To Dr. Shannon and the health4life family – It's Just 12 Weeks!

To the Dynamic Sports Development Team – Are You Ready for The Next Level?

To my awesome production team-1260 Productions.com and my editor Jamie Fithian- Thank You!

To Rocco, "The King of Branding," Thank you for the late night coaching phone calls and for bringing clarity to my brand.

To everyone who I have not mentioned, who has crossed my

path and impacted me in some way to be better in life, I say thank you!

There are so many people to thank – I could write a whole book of thank you's.

Most of all, I want to thank YOU! This book was written for you, and without you there would be no book.

Thank you

Jonathan Conneely "Coach JC"

CONTENTS

WHAT IS THE SECRET TO REAL WEIGHT LOSS SUCCESS

Do you want to live with the pain of discipline or the pain
of regret? The pain of discipline lasts a short amount of
time while the pain of regret lasts a lifetime!

Before you start this book, I need to address two very important factors:

RETENTION WITHOUT IMPLEMENTATION IS USELESS!

In this book, within the next 27 chapters, you will receive life-changing information, or should I say, potentially life–changing information. How many times have you started a book and not completed it? On the other hand, maybe you have read many books, but your life seems to stay the same. Believe me, you are not the only one!

Why is this? Retention with implementation! In this book you are going to receive the necessary tools to take your life to the next level. You are going to receive the real truth to your fat loss that you have long been awaiting. I want to caution that you must put this valuable information into play for it to work for you. Retention without implementation will not do you any good. While reading this book, if you begin to implement these valuable tactics on a daily basis, you will become a "new person" who will literally be able to do whatever you want to do and accomplish true success. So I must say it again: do yourself a favor and please do not allow this to be just another book. Instead, allow it to be the book that changes your life forever! That is exactly what Jessica decided to do!

"Before starting Coach JC's Bootcamp Tulsa Program
I had completely let myself go. I gave birth to my son
and couldn't get all of the baby weight off. I dis-liked
my tummy most of all and had absolutely no energy, I

had 100% become lazy. I was so scared of not making it
through that first workout and looking silly. I just figured
since I couldn't commit to a gym or a diet, I would give
Bootcamp Tulsa a shot. Since training with Coach JC, I
have lost 16 pounds, 12 inches and went from a size 12
to a tight size 8! I love the way I feel about myself, My
self-confidence has increased as I watch my body firm
and tighten, and I have more energy then I know what to
do with. I admire Coach JC's style of training for many
reasons. When you have a coach who can inspire change,
build a teamwork environment, and hold you accountable
for the commitment you have made to yourself, that, to
me, is AMAZING!

Transform YOUR life!

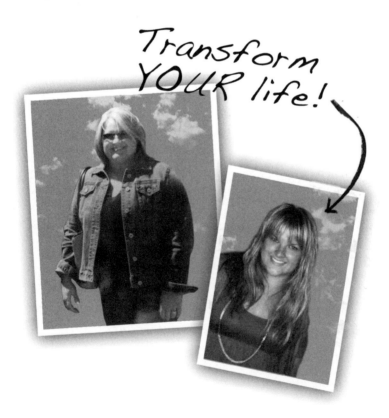

He is inspiring and the passion seeps out of him with every comment he makes. Coach JC truly loves transforming lives. Now, I'm happy with myself and the results I have seen in just Ten Weeks! I feel more productive, and I have been able to inspire change in others around me, especially after beating my husband in push-ups! I never thought I would form an addiction to working out, but I absolutely look forward to those days now. I'm excited to see what the future training will do for my mind, body, and spirit."

Jessica Mathias — 29 years old

WHY YOU SHOULD FINISH THIS BOOK!

There are a number of reasons why you should finish this book. First of all, it is great training. If you keep quitting one thing and going onto another, you will never get anywhere. Too many quitters live in the world today! Even if you don't use all of the knowledge right away, there will come a time in the future when you will need it. Preparation time is never wasted time!

This is one great reason, but I also want to notify you about another important reason for sticking with this book until the end. Each of the chapters, especially the Game Plan in chapter 27, are delivered systematically, and in sequential order, so that you can act on them immediately and start seeing the results that you deserve.

This means that if you decide not to finish until some point in the future, you will need to start all over with the very first chapter to see the most optimal results.

I strongly encourage you to allow these next 27 chapters to change your life forever! Trust me when I say that you will thank me in the end.

This is not just another book; it is a game plan — a plan of action, a call to greatness – to help you learn how to take control of your life and to actually live out those things that you always dreamed.

Some of the chapters that you come across will be uncomfortable. That is too bad! You may think that you do not need some of the things in this book. I want to tell you: do not be fooled, if you are serious about taking control of your life, then now is the time to set your pride aside and let this book transform you for good.

Also, please understand that timing is everything. It is not a mistake that you chose this book at this time in your life. This is the right time and this is the right book for you. This book contains the plan of action for which you have been seeking. Now is your time! It is time to devote the next 27 days to a new you! Yes, just 27 days! Are you willing?

Now, if you are ready, let's get to the real reason why you are here… the next level awaits you!!

J. Conneely

Jonathan Conneely

"Coach JC"

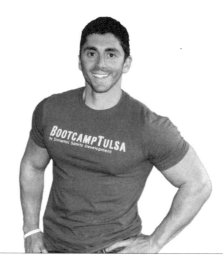

MEET YOUR PERSONAL COACH!

Hi, my name is Jonathan Conneely "Coach JC" and I am your coach! I have been assisting individuals from all walks of life to "take it to the next level!" I love to motivate people to take control of their lives by taking control of their health. I have a great passion for helping people live their lives to the fullest. I received my bachelor's degree in Health and Exercise Science, and I am a certified SCCc Strength Coach. I am the Founder and President of the well recognized Sports Performance Company, Dynamic Sports Development. I also founded Bootcamp Tulsa, Tulsa's first–ever outdoor fitness program. In addition, I am the Director of Strength and Conditioning at an NCAA Division I institution and the developer of the Health4life Transformation Challenge. My coaching philosophy is simple: I am dedicated to providing the tools necessary to empower individuals to create ultimate lifestyle changes.

I am a native of New Jersey and have been residing in Tulsa, Oklahoma since 1999. I am actively involved member of the Tulsa community, and I am also an active member of the best church in the world, Victory Christian Center. I love people and want to see people live a fulfilled, happy, and healthy life! You can learn more about me and what I do at CoachJC.com

I must tell you that I do not look at this as a book, but rather as a coaching program. I am a coach, and I coach people for a living. That is who I am, what I do, and what I love to do. What do you think of when you hear the word, "coach?" You probably think of a football or basketball coach, someone who instructs athletes in a sport. That is true to some extent, but I believe a coach is something even more.

A Coach?

I believe that a coach is a person who possesses and uses the necessary tools, knowledge, and wisdom to elicit a client's values, goals, and beliefs, so that together they can create strategies and a plan of action for success in the client's life. A coach is a model for success! He or she does this by demonstrating balance in his or her own life. An effective and successful coach creates a relationship of trust and respect, while still offering the truth, regardless of whether it is good or bad. That is what I will be doing in this book – I Will Be Your Coach!

What is Coaching?

To be successful, the coach must be able to create and maintain a connection of safety and trust between himself and the client. Once that is established, the coach can proceed to create conditions of excellence and strategies of action so that the client can achieve the results they desire. So, congratulations, you now have your very own, personal coach! Go and tell your friends! I am your coach, and throughout this book, I will be coaching you.

I train athletes for a living, and I am a health and wellness professional. Throughout my career, I have seen the athlete, who had all the talent in the world, go on and never achieve ultimate success. I have also seen the kid, who most people thought would never make it, go on to achieve great success in their respective sport. Why is this? Well, I truly believe that over the last ten years of coaching I have figured out the secret. In this book,

I am going to reveal that secret to you by coaching you to success. I am also going to give you the tools and the key things you must do in order to walk in ultimate success and have whatever it is that you desire.

Why do some people lose weight but eventually put it back on? Why do some athletes never achieve peak performance in their sports? Why do some athletes never get to experience the highest level while others do? Why do some people make more money than others? Why do some people go through life feeling like they are not achieving what they are here on earth to achieve? It is all because they are not coachable! Are you coachable? I do not believe in the easy way out. However, I do believe that you can work all day, putting the time in, but still never reach the highest level if you do not possess the keys to success. To be your best, you must possess those keys and you must be willing to be coached. In this book, I am going to give you those keys. The question is, are you coachable? By the way, this is the least expensive coaching session that you could ever receive. Make the most of it!

WHAT TO EXPECT IN THIS COACHING PROGRAM

In this book, I am going to systematically deliver to you the truth about what it takes to lose the weight that you always desired to lose. I am going to give you the real secret behind how you can look and feel the way that you always dreamed of.

I will be giving you real life concepts on how you can step into ultimate success and how you can have whatever you want as soon as you choose to have it. This book is going to be your plan of action, your game plan. Please realize that all successful game plans take practice to execute properly, and this sometimes is a process. The first part of the process is understanding the true reason of why you want what you want. This is also the most important part of the process. A foundation is essential for any new game plan to be executed properly. The foundation here is – Why do you want what it is that you want?

Before you read another page in this book you need to know the answer to that question!

At the conclusion of this book, you will:

- Have all the tools necessary to achieve the body that you have always desired.

- Look and feel great about yourself!

- Be healthier and live a more abundant life.

- Have the mindset that will allow you to have anything that you want, any time that you want it.

- Understand what it really takes to get fit and how simple it really can be.

- Anticipate the future that lies ahead of you, and truly know what it is that you deserve.

- Understand the real keys to losing weight for good!

- Understand the true secret to fat loss that no one else wants to tell you.

- Understand what you need to do in order to take control of your life for good.

- Have the same game plan that has produced life-changing results in thousands of people's lives.

- Have the motivation to build your life the way you want to build it.

- Be able to conquer those things in your life that you have always desired.

Let me ask you…

What does ultimate freedom mean to you? What does true health look like to you? What does ultimate success look like to you? Now, let me change the question – if you had all the freedom in the world that you could want, what would you be doing right now?

What if you could just get up in the morning and know that you can provide for yourself and for your family? What if you could obtain the fitness level that you desire? What if you could finally achieve the body that you have always wished for? What if you could finally have those things of which you have always dreamed, and what if you could have those things whenever you want and however you want?

Freedom is an attitude and all of us have a different idea of the true definition of freedom.

I want you to understand one thing from this book, and that is this:

No matter where you are currently at in your life, today can be the start of a new beginning! Whatever that thing is that you desire so badly, you can have it if you simply take the time to learn how to get it. In this coaching program, I am going to give you the necessary keys so that you can experience freedom in your life.

This book is going to provide you with the knowledge on how to go and get it!

WHY THIS BOOK WAS CREATED

This book was created because I am sick and tired of people not living their life to the fullest. I want to help you revolutionize your life so that you can walk out what you are called to do on this earth. I wrote this book with you in mind. I know that you are capable of great things! Yes, in life there are struggles and you will face obstacles, but you are still capable of having whatever you want, whenever you want it. The question is, how badly do you really want that thing or things? If you want it badly enough then you can have it!

WHAT THIS BOOK IS NOT

This book is not just another fitness book or workout book that is going to provide you with a cookie–cutter workout. This book is definitely not just another diet book; we all know how much everyone loves to diet.

You have probably seen hundreds of infomercials, advertisements, and book after book about losing weight, cutting unwanted body fat, and obtaining six–pack abs. You may have even purchased these products or ordered these magazines. Are you the person that always buys the latest diet book or workout DVD? Let me state once again, that this is not just another diet book. This is not just another book to get you pumped up and excited to lose some weight. This book is about way more than that. This book is about your life; this book will transform your life forever. That is, if you want it to, and if you allow it to. This is your personal coaching program. You will receive a game plan with the most effective fat–burning exercise routines, along with nutritional coaching and recommendations. If you want to lose weight, increase strength, become healthier, and see results in your physique, then this book is for you. If you want to have anything that you want any time that you want it, this book is for you!

This book is more then just about losing weight and looking good, this book is about your life. I am going to give you the necessary principles for you to accomplish the body transformation that you desire. The workout contains some of the most effective routines that have worked for thousands of people. The nutrition coaching is simple and effective and has been life-changing for thousands of people. However, one more part of the game plan makes it complete, and that is the content in the chapters leading up to the game plan. So, for you to be successful at this, your game plan starts right now!

Are you ready to lose those extra pounds and know that you can keep the weight off for good?

Are you sick and tired of losing weight and putting it back on?

Are you sick and tired of all the empty promises out there?

Are you sick and tired of not being able to live your best life?

What if you could live your best life with the body that you have always desired?

Would you want that?

Good, then you are at the right place! After you are done with these 27 days, you will not have to go searching for the magic pill any longer, you will not have to purchase another piece of equipment or DVD from an infomercial ever again. I understand that losing the weight is an important part of your life and that is why you bought this book in the first place. You will lose that weight and experience the physical results that you desire, but please understand that what I am talking about here is a total transformation! I am not talking about losing a few pounds and then putting those same pounds (and more) back on next month. For many people, losing the weight is not the hardest part. Instead, trying to keep it off is when people struggle to succeed. You have probably have a friend, a family member, or even yourself who has been in this situation. Why is this? You are about to find out! I am talking about making a lifestyle change that will revolutionize not only the way you look, but also the way you feel and the WAY YOU THINK! You have probably heard the proverb, what a man thinketh, he is. I am not talking about a quick fix, but a lifestyle makeover! This is not just about losing the stubborn weight now but about losing it forever! I get numerous emails on a daily basis from people who just can't understand why they cannot experience the body that they want. Is there some kind of secret? Maybe you are one of these people who have tried it all and just don't understand why you can't achieve what you want.

So what is that secret? The secret is… **The Power of the Mind!**

Are you serious? That is it – the power of the mind? That is right! Those people who never achieve what they desire and deserve is simply because they don't possess the right mindset! That athlete who does not achieve the highest level? It is because of his mindset! That person who does not live financially free? Mindset! That person who cannot lose the weight they desire? Mindset! That person who loses the weight and then puts it right back on? Mindset!

Okay, first let me clarify something. Talent and skill are a must! I say this because I have seen some people with the right mindset never do big things simply because they did not possess the skill or the talent in that area. So, don't let me mislead you into thinking that you can just have the right mindset and have anything that you want. We will speak more about this later.

This book was born out of my experiences from training athletes on all levels, consulting people of all occupations, and also from my own experiences. I get asked all the time, what did you do to be so successful at such a young age? Believe me, I am not even close to where I want to be and not even close to fulfilling what my purpose is on this earth. However, I can tell you that I have applied the mindset principles that you will learn in this book to my own life and that they work. I made a decision years ago that I was going to do whatever it took to be successful. I can honestly tell you that the combination of my skill and talent, along with these principles is what made me successful. Now understand, success is measured differently by everyone. For me, it was to be prosperous in a few certain areas. I wanted to be spiritually stable, financially established, and physically healthy. I believed that if I could possess success in those areas, then I would have the freedom to fulfill what I was called to do on this earth.

I want you to know that the keys and steps that I am about to share with you are simple and easy to follow. These principles will work for anyone! If you have not realized it yet, you are holding the book with the necessary tools for you to experience ultimate success in your life! You are going to have the keys to accomplishing anything that you want, any time that you want! You are about to be educated and empowered to take back what is yours! That body that you have been wanting for over 20 years, you can now have it!

You are holding this book, at this time in your life, for a special reason and for a special purpose. I want you to realize that...

Now is Your Time!

Maybe your doctor told you that you need to take control of your health, maybe you just need to feel good again, maybe you need to lose 200 pounds, maybe you want to lose 20 pounds, maybe you want to take control of your life, maybe you just want to be healthy, or maybe you are just sick and tired of being sick and tired. I have great news for you! Now you can have any and all of those things. The principles in this book will give you the freedom to experience ultimate success!

I have implemented these same 27 keys into my own life, and I can tell you that they work! I know they have worked for me and my life because of my faith. I am at the level I am today because of these principles, but my faith in Jesus Christ has also played a large role. This 27–day program will work, and you will see great results. You will be motivated, you will lose weight, and you will have success in your life; however, if you want the ultimate results and the ultimate success, then I encourage you to get your life right with Christ. The power I have experienced in the Word of God has been life–changing for me. I can honestly say that I would not be where I am today if it were not for my relationship with Jesus Christ.

Before we start this transformation, I want to tell you that He is a good God and can do the same great things for you if you allow him. It is a simple process: you can accept Jesus as your LORD and Savior right now, right where you are. Please visit Victory.com; this is the website for my home church. The people there will take care of you and lead you in the right direction. My pastor at Victory, Billy Joe Daugherty, has been a huge inspiration to me and the writing of this book. I want you to know that even with the perfect body, all the money in the world, and unlimited success, you will never feel content or fulfilled without a personal faith in Jesus Christ.

I am excited for you and for the next 27 days! Let's get started!

WARNING!

Now, I must warn you that if you apply the Secret To Real Weight Loss Success principles, your life will never be the same. Your life will be drastically changed forever! Your family and friends may not even recognize you after awhile. Strangers will be stopping you on the street wondering what it is that you do and what you have that they do not.

Are you ready for this?

Now, I also must caution you that some of the things I say may anger and even frustrate you. My approach is very blunt and stern. People in America die every day because of health–related diseases. I cannot sit around and watch this happen when I know that this book contains the key to life and death.

I wrote this book because of a hurting heart. My heart hurts to see people who aren't happy with the way they look and then to see this unhappiness filter into other areas of their lives. My heart hurts to see people living life at 50% of what they should be. My heart hurts to see the obese children of America. My heart hurts to see people who are not experiencing happiness in their lives. I have developed such a passion for this topic that it burns inside of me. This book is 10 years of hands–on experience, 10 years of research, and 10 years in the making, and at least 15 years of heart ache!

We are not promised tomorrow and we never know what the future has in store. So please understand that I am very passionate about what I do and that I am a straight shooter – I will say it how it is. We are going to have a relationship similar to the one you had with your high school sweetheart. There may be times in this book when you get angry and frustrated at me and wonder, "How could he say that?" But believe me, when you have completed this game plan and your life has been transformed, you are going to look back and thank me. You will thank me for delivering the information that you needed to hear and that no one else was going to tell you. It's that love/hate relationship: hate me one moment, yet love me the next – just like your high school romance.

I want you to understand something: I did not write this book to make you feel good but to motivate and challenge you to make yourself better. Sometimes the truth hurts, but it is that truth that will ultimately set you free.

When I tell you that you will never have to start another fad diet again, I mean that. When I tell you that you will not have to search the Internet to find the latest miracle fat loss pill ever again, I mean that. When I tell you that you will never have to feel like a failure again, I mean that. This will be the last book you will ever need in regards to changing your body and losing weight. This will be the last book you will ever need to purchase to show you how to lose excess body fat and look and feel good again. If you want this to be, it will be the last time you need to feel like you don't have control of your life. This book will do it for you, but only if you do it for yourself!

In this book, I am going to show you how once you conquer your thinking, it will lead not only to great weight loss, but also to a lifestyle change to keep that weight off for good and to help conquer other areas of your life.

The power of the mind is the key to your success, and you can have that success today!

Let me repeat, if you are looking for a quick fix, this is not the book for you.

I am going to give you a step-by-step approach on how to conquer your mindset. A 27-day game plan to take your life back for good! I am going to show you how to lose weight, how to do it the right way, and how to keep it off for good!

If you want this to be the last time that you are
not happy with your body... Keep reading!

If you never want to go searching for that
magical fat loss pill again... Keep Reading!

If you want your life to be not just good, but
great ... Keep Reading!

If you are sick and tired of not seeing the results
that you desire... Keep reading!

*You deserve those results and now is the time
to take back what you deserve*

...Your Health and Your Life!

Before we start, I want you to hear from one of my clients who has changed her life forever by using the same tools that you will be receiving in this coaching program!

"Before joining Coach JC's program, I was not moti-

vated to stick to an exercise regimen. I would workout

on my own here and there, but not regularly. I was also

only walking or running and not strength training, so I

was not in great shape muscularly. I was skeptical about

training with Coach JC's program because I didn't know if I could keep up. Since I had never truly "trained" before, I was afraid of failure. That fear was totally unfounded, though, because Coach JC will always work with you at your level, and then help you to increase your ability to push to the NEXT level.

I have seen tremendous results while training with Coach JC! I have lost weight and body fat and have increased my physical strength and ability 100%. I have been a part of the Bootcamp Tulsa family for over a year, and even after the first month, I saw dramatic results. That is why I have continued to be a repeat customer!

What I love about Coach JC's style of training is that he is very motivational. He genuinely cares about the individual's fitness goals and about people in general. He gets to know you personally. He takes the time to ask you personalized questions to help him in determining what changes you may need to make to gain the most benefit from your training. Even when working out on my own, I hear Coach JC's voice in my head 'GET THERE! Finish Strong! Rep It Out!'

What I would say to someone who gets the opportunity to train with Coach JC would be: DO IT!!! Stop procrastinating. Stop making excuses as to why you can't get into shape. Just give him a chance to prove to you that you CAN do it! Lots of other people have been successful, and if they can do it, so can you! It's not easy.

Nothing in life worth having is easy, but the rewards of getting healthy and being in shape are priceless!

While doing the full program, I lost a total of seven percent of my body fat! My life now is much more healthy. I have gotten an education about what is healthy to eat and about the proper way to workout. I feel GREAT, because I am staying active and living life to the fullest! Thanks Coach JC!"

Tasa Proberts — 37 years old

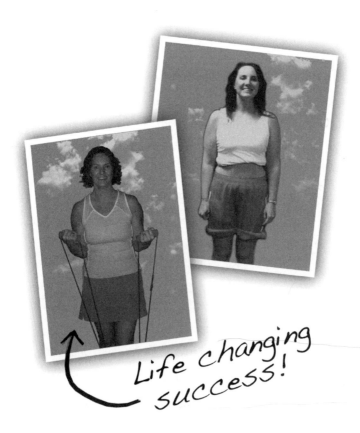

Life changing success!

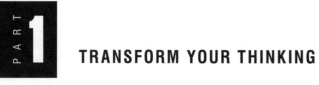

PART 1

TRANSFORM YOUR THINKING

CHAPTER ONE

DISCOVER THE 3 KEYS TO SUCCESS

How blessed is the man who finds wisdom,
and the man who gains understanding.

Proverbs 3:13

YOU MUST WANT IT!

To be successful in any area of your life, I believe that you must possess three components.

The first key component is **desire**. You must have a desire for what it is you want to do. You must have a desire for what you want to accomplish. For you to have invested money to purchase this book and to have read this much already, shows me that you have the desire. You have the desire to lose that unwanted body fat! You have the desire for change! You have the desire to be successful! Having that desire is a must, but that desire is not enough. It takes more than that. Think about it: a lot of people in the world desire to be millionaires, but how many of those people actually become millionaires? A lot of people desire to look good physically and live a healthy lifestyle, but how many people really experience that to the fullest? A lot of people, like you, desire to lose weight and unwanted body fat, but how many people really see the results they desire? I hope you understand the point that desire is not enough; just wanting it will not get it for you. However, you must want it!

Understand that desire is the first component you must possess and if you don't have it, the rest of the steps will not function the correct way. Without a true desire you will eventually fail. I am not going to sit here and tell you that this is going to be easy. If losing weight were easy, you would have seen the results you desire and would not even be reading this book right now. It is going to take hard work and some discipline. It is going to take consistency and sweat. Times are going to be tough and the road is not always going to be paved. When you have that desire – that burning desire – it will push you through those times.

So as you can see, desire is a must. You have to want it; you have to desire it!

What is it that you want? What is it that you so badly desire?

HOW MUCH DO YOU REALLY KNOW?

The second component that you must possess is **knowledge**. You have probably heard the saying that people perish for the lack of knowledge. I believe this to be very true. For example, if you want to be a millionaire, you have to have some knowledge on how to make a million dollars. You can have all the desire in the world to be a millionaire, but without the knowledge, it will be hard to acquire that much money (unless of course you inherit it or win the lottery). Even then, you must possess some knowledge on how to make that money work for you and how to turn it into five million dollars. How many times do you hear about someone winning the lottery and then losing all of the money within a few months? That makes me sick.

The same thing applies to losing weight; you must have knowledge about what to do to lose the weight, but also to keep it off. What kind of exercising is best for accomplishing your goal? What do you need to eat on a regular basis? These are just some of the questions you will need to answer. For example, you must have some knowledge on the proper technique and form of exercise and how much to do. The great thing about this book is that I am going to give you this knowledge. I will give you the right tools and the right knowledge to be successful. You can have some knowledge on how to make a million dollars, but if it is the wrong knowledge or information, you are just wasting your time. Now you can have the peace of mind to know that you will have the right knowledge and information. What I will do in this book is give you some knowledge in regard to the right exercises to perform and the right nutrients to take in, but most importantly, I want to give you some knowledge on how to change your thinking. This will ultimately lead you to the promise land of not only losing that weight but also keeping it off for good.

Now, let me pose a quick question: with all the books, CDs, DVDs, gyms, and miscellaneous information on health and weight loss, why are we still a country of obese people? Why are so many people not seeing the results they desire? Why is child-hood obesity on the rise? Why are people sometimes losing the weight but then putting it right back on? Well, that is where the third component becomes important.

YOU MUST HAVE A GAME PLAN!

To be successful, you must have a plan of action – a game plan! I believe that this is the area where most people fail. Those individuals who have the desire and the knowledge to make a million dollars, still need to have a plan of action. Look at any sports team from an eight–year–old team to a professional team; they all have a game plan. Like the saying goes, if you fail to plan, then you are planning to fail! So, what I want to give you in this book, is a step–by–step plan of action – a game plan! You have probably read several books that give you all this in-formation, but they never give you a plan of action on how to implement it. It is like the ultimate suspense movie with 30 min-utes left, and then the power goes out. You were almost there and bam! You probably asked yourself: where do I go from here or where do I begin? That is one of the reasons why I wrote this book: to give you a plan of action, and to give you the tools necessary to thrive. Now, in order for this plan to work, you must follow it step–by–step. Some of you will get anxious and will want to skip ahead. That is fine if you want to go and take a look, but for you to get the ultimate results, you must follow the plan in order. Every game plan has a systematic sequence to it, as does this one. Sure, you can skip over the transform your thinking part and just perform the workout. You will see some results because the workout is that good, but I am not interested

TRANSFORM YOUR THINKING

in you seeing some results, and I am not interested in you living a mediocre life. I want you to accomplish all of your goals and live the best, healthiest, most fulfilled life that you can. If you just want to be good then maybe this isn't the book for you; however, if you are ready to be GREAT then it is time to discover The Secret To Real Weight Loss Success!

Let the fun begin!

CHAPTER TWO

DISCOVER THE POWER OF THE MIND

Once you conquer your mind, you conquer your life

So many people today never accomplish what they want to in life or what they were called to do simply because they allow their minds to hold them back. You can probably think of a situation where you knew that you should have done something but didn't act simply because mentally you would not allow yourself to it. In this chapter, I am going to give you a few things that have to change in order for you to accomplish your goals. We are not just going to talk about how to change your thinking in regard to weight loss. This book is about changing your thinking... period!

You will be surprised that when you change a habit in your thinking on to lose weight, other areas in your life will be affected. You will see your marriage and personal relationships go to a whole other level. You will see that your whole demeanor will improve and your business will explode. Why is this? There is a filtering effect. Once you learn how to conquer the way that you think, you will see that this new mindset will affect many areas in your entire life, areas that you did not even plan on improving. Maybe you have a spouse, a friend, or a family member who is not succeeding in a certain area of his or her life. She can apply these same principles for that area of her life and transform her life forever. That is the whole reason why I addressed this book in the way that I did. I want to see people walk out their destiny! Your health is just one area; you losing weight is just one area. I want to see you live a prosperous life. I want you to live life to the fullest in every area. You can lose the desired weight and still not be happy and prosperous in life! A lot of times when I say prosperous people automatically think I am talking about financially. To me, financial success is only one area of being prosperous in life. How many times have you seen a rich person who is very unhappy? If you have all the money in the world, but you are miserable and sick, you are not living a prosperous life. You can be the most fit–looking person in America, but if your marriage and other relationships are struggling, then you are not living a prosperous life. You could have great health and a great family situation but struggling just to pay the monthly bills; that is also not living in prosperity. To me, prosperous is being successful in all areas of your life: health, finances, spiritual and mental. So my point is, be ready for other areas of your life, besides just your physical appearance, to take a turn in the positive direction.

Now is the time to chase your dreams! I want you to hear from one of my very special clients who had the desire for change in her life and chased that dream.

Check out these amazing results!
Hillary lost 30 pounds and dropped 4 dress sizes.

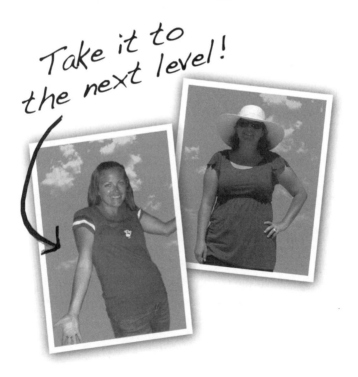

Take it to the next level!

*Coach JC and Bootcamp Tulsa have changed my life!
I knew that I needed to start getting active again but I
was scared to death to put myself out there. One day I
saw Coach JC on our local news and I thought to myself,
"That is what I need." Like most of us, I had to "think"
about it. A couple of days later Bootcamp Tulsa popped
up on my Facebook and I knew it was meant to be, so I
signed up.*

*I was so SCARED to go the first day!!! But I went
and thank goodness I did! Coach JC and Bootcamp Tulsa
were just the right tools I needed for me to lose weight.
The motivation I received from Coach JC's program
helped me succeed in reaching my goals of becoming a
healthier and happier ME. You cannot put a price or
words for the way I feel about myself now and the grati-
tude I have towards Coach JC and Bootcamp Tulsa for
giving me the tools to transform my life.*

*Within five months of starting Coach JC's program
I have lost 30 pounds and have dropped four dress
sizes!!!!! The program has taught me how to exercise
correctly and to make healthier eating choices. I'm at
the point in my life that I want to workout, I want to be
healthy, I want a better me and I want to step out of my
box and experience life. All of these life changing experiences I've encountered over the last five months are all
because I followed and listened to Coach JC's program.
Thanks Coach!!!!!*

Hillary Pritchard – 30 years old

TRANSFORM YOUR THINKING

1

CHAPTER THREE

DO DREAM BIG

I have been called a dreamer my whole life…
this book was once just a dream. Nothing will
happen unless you first dream!

I ask people all the time, what does your dream body look like? Some people explain to me this great body – the one you would see on a fitness magazine cover, while others just express that it would be weighing 20 pounds less. Still others express that it would be having 10 to 15 pounds of more muscle. My next question is, if that is your dream body, then why don't you look like that? Most of the responses are, "Oh that's not possible!" or "That's not realistic!" It always makes me laugh. I am amazed at how many people just don't dream big. Then there are people that dream big but never chase those dreams. You need to not only dream but also go and make those dreams a reality. A dream without action will always just be a dream. Put some action behind those dreams and the sky is the limit.

If you want to lose weight, I am not telling you to just sit there and dream of losing weight. Believe me, you won't lose weight by just sitting there! What I am telling you is that if you want to lose weight, you must dream big, you must see that image of yourself losing weight on a daily basis, you must see that image of you succeeding. You must see the final product! Believe, without a doubt, that your dream will come to past and don't quit believing. I am not talking about living in denial. I am talking about believing and going out and doing it. It is time to chase those dreams! Don't see yourself any more as being fat; instead, begin to claim that dream. Don't see yourself any more as being unhealthy; go chase it! Once you complete this book, you will have learned how to make that dream a true reality, but first, you must develop a mental picture of what you will look like.

Make this picture as definite and specific as possible. Remember what it is that you desire and never let that get clouded. If this is truly what you desire, this is the picture you must continually have in your mind: the image of what you will look like when you get there. You need to know what it is that you want and you need to want it so badly that it will stay in your thoughts on a constant basis. Once you have that dream, once you see this picture, there is one more thing that you must do. You must ask yourself: what is the purpose? Why do you really want to lose this weight? Do you want to look better? Do you want to feel better about yourself? Do you want to live longer and live free of disease? It is this purpose that will continually drive you. A dream without a purpose will just be a dream. The purpose is what will drive you; the purpose is what is going to keep you motivated; the purpose is what is going to make this dream, this mental picture, become tangible.

Dream Big!

TRANSFORM YOUR THINKING

1

CHAPTER FOUR

DON'T MAKE EXCUSES

What's more important: your excuse or your motive?

So many people have excuse after excuse for why they are not achieving what they desire. You have to change that mindset. Make a decision that starting today, in all that you do, you will not make excuses for any part of it. How many times do you hear people say, "because of my parents I am…" or "because of my spouse I am…?" Have you ever listened to someone speak and all they talk about is how nothing is their fault, including the incidents and actions that put them in the situation that they are in? It is time to take responsibility for your life. Don't blame our society for the reason why you are not fit. Yes, that is a big problem, with all of the fast food and junk food and the marketing that goes with it, but you aren't forced to eat it. You are the one that ultimately purchases it and eats it.

I also hear this excuse all of the time, "Oh, I can't lose weight because of my body type; I have bad genetics." Yes, there are some true reasons that people cannot lose weight, but instead of making excuses, you should be grateful that you are not one of those people. Some situations like thyroid issues and other diseases that restrict weight loss need to be treated by a physician and should be taken seriously. If that is not your case, then it is time to take responsibility for your physical appearance and to stop making excuses. This is such a powerful thing because without it you will look at your life as a failure and never accomplish your dreams and goals. Once you take responsibility, you will begin to experience peace and joy and control over every circumstance. You must begin to understand that you are ultimately responsible for your choices, which should be a great feeling. A feeling of CONTROL! To me, this is a great feeling – to know that your life is your responsibility and that no one can

live your life for you. You are in charge! This is your life! Even
when events that are not under your control go wrong, you can
at least determine how you will react to the event. This is where
you can choose to make the event a disaster or use it to make
you better. I want you to begin to use it as an opportunity to
learn and to grow. Maybe you have made mistakes in life, but
guess what? We all have, but from here on out that is the past.
Starting today, you need to take responsibility for where you are
currently, and tomorrow, begin to look ahead and not look back.
Blaming yourself for the past won't do anything but hold you
back from your future.

No More Excuses!

TRANSFORM YOUR THINKING

1

CHAPTER FIVE

DECIDE TO LET NEGATIVITY GO

Negativity is like cancer, it will eventually kill you!

We have become a society filled with negativity. Everywhere you turn, everything is negative this and negative that. Turn on the TV or the news and what do you hear? We are bombarded on a daily basis with negative situations. A large part of you changing your thinking is eliminating those negative sources in your life. First of all, you must eliminate any negativity that you think about yourself. Maybe it is "I am fat, I am unhealthy, I will always be poor, or I am no good, etc.." Now, I am not saying that you should live in denial; I am talking about how you view yourself. You were wonderfully made and created for a purpose and it is time to fulfill that purpose. You were born a winner, but over time the world has taught you to fail and has planted negativity in your mind. You need to begin to identify those negative patterns and address them by eliminating them on a daily basis. Then you must begin to eliminate the negative outside sources. Sometimes this is very hard because it could be a close friend or even a family member. Maybe a loved one has told you that you won't be successful, that you won't amount to much, that you are not beautiful, or that you can't lose weight. Words are a powerful tool and you can really begin to believe these things and your life may reflect it. Well, I have good news for you! Today is the day of new beginnings for you, the day of change. It is time to draw a line in the sand and take a stand that you will no longer accept this negativity in your life. If you can't completely remove yourself from this negativity, then you need to begin to close your ears when you are around those people. I don't mean stuff toilet paper in your ears; I am talking about blanking them out. You can choose what you are exposed to. When things become negative, change the subject or if necessary, leave the room. This is your life, so take control of it today! This next part is hard for people to do and that is to limit your exposure to the media. Every time you turn on the news, negativity. Every time you pick up the paper, negativity. Every time you turn on the radio, negativity. I am amazed at how many people listen and read this garbage on a daily basis. People are religiously feeding on this media soap opera, which is packed with negativity and gossip. Besides being negative, this crap is also a time robber. Think about how much time you spend watching TV or reading that garbage. You could invest some of that time getting one step closer to your weight loss goal. This is so powerful, and some people just don't get it. I am telling you that if you are around negativity, you will become negative in many different areas of your life. You have to make the decision to disassociate yourself with these things. Do not listen to media that portrays this negative mentally; do not associate with people who are always negative. Get rid of the magazines and books that portray this dark gossip.

Eliminate the garbage in your life!

TRANSFORM YOUR THINKING

1

CHAPTER SIX

DETERMINE YOUR ATTITUDE

If you don't like something, change
it; if you can't change it, change the
way you think about it.

Mary Engelbreit

Your attitude is a lot more important than you think. Everyone knows people who have a bad attitude. Do you really enjoy being around those people? Some characteristics must be a part of your attitude in order for you to be successful and live life to the fullest.

A lot of people just sit around and feel sorry for themselves. Where you are today is a direct correlation to what you did yesterday. If you don't like where you are at in your life – what job you have, your physical appearance, or how much you weigh – only one person can change that and that is you. You have to take that attitude of feeling sorry for yourself and transform it into something positive. Quit worrying about where you are at currently and focus on where you want to be.

Your attitude reflects who you are; what is on the inside is what comes out.

Today, I want you to start to develop an attitude, but not the kind that you are thinking about. I am talking about your outlook of who you are, about your perception of what you can really accomplish, about your mindset of getting back into shape, about taking a stance for what you want, and about having the attitude of achieving what you ultimately need and deserve... a happy, prosperous life! It is time to change your attitude! Do you know that there are countless people who will never reach their destiny and ultimate health until you achieve yours? Yes, there are others who depend upon you. There is a much larger picture involved. I created this coaching program not only so you could transform your life, but also so you can make everyone who you are associated with better. That is what life is really about! It's time for you to change your attitude and begin to know that anything you want to accomplish you can have. Begin to know that the results you desire will come! Develop the attitude of "who cares how long it takes, I will not quit until I get there." Begin to no longer look at where you are, but began to see where you are going. Start to change your attitude now, knowing that your desired body is right around the corner. Start to walk with a confidence, not cockiness, but a confidence that no one can get in your way, no one can prevent you from seeing those life-changing results, no one can steal your dream to look good and feel good about yourself again.

Get A Little Attitude!

TRANSFORM YOUR THINKING

1

CHAPTER SEVEN

DON'T ACCEPT FAILURE

*If you don't fear failing, it is because you
never started anything!*

Failure is not an option! If you believe that you are going to fail, then you will fail. Think about it: it took Thomas Edison over 1,000 attempts to create the light bulb. Now, that is a no-quit attitude! Imagine if he had quit! Today and from here on out, you will establish the no-quit mentality – the no-quit attitude. You have probably tried diet after diet, personal trainer after personal trainer, infomercial product after infomercial product. You may have spent a lot of time and money on all of these things but over and over have come up short. You may feel as if you have failed. You may even look at yourself as a failure in this specific area. Starting today, I want you to focus on having a no-quit attitude.

From here on out, I want you to give yourself permission to fail. In my coaching program, failure does not really exist, but with this permission, you will figure out ways not to do it. So many people try the newest thing until the next newest thing comes along. Today, I want you to promise yourself that you are going to get through this entire coaching program, that you are going to finish. So many people worry about what is going to happen if it doesn't work, and then fear sets in and they jump to the next thing. You must see the program through to completion. If it works or if it doesn't work, you will feel good that you finished something. Here is the cool thing: this program is set up so you don't fail. It works! This program won't fail you. The only way it won't work is if you fail it. Now, once you promise yourself that you are going to finish, you must finish. That may mean getting up earlier to make sure that you get the workout in. That may mean pushing yourself to make sure that you get the workout completed. These small steps will go a long way, and eventually you will begin to see yourself conquering this area of your life. This will build momentum and you will begin to see success. This success will lead to more focus and will lead to success in another area of your life.

Start to think big! What if you could lose that extra 20 pounds, what if you could make an extra $50 thousand a year, what if your marriage could be the best? Start to allow your vision to expand. Take the pressure off yourself; what is the worst thing that is going to happen? The answer is you will see your life take a turn in the right direction. Finish what you start! I am going to make it easy for you by giving you a day-by-day game plan. This way you are going to have a deadline. It always helps when you give yourself a deadline.

So many people never start anything because they are so worried about the outcome, so worried about failing. I tend to look at it differently: if you never start, you have already failed.

Get Started!

I tried for many years to lose weight; I spent endless hours in the gym and thousands of dollars on personal training. I thought that if I worked out for hours every day that I could lose the weight that I wanted. I subscribed to all the fitness magazines because I desperately wanted to look and feel good about myself again. Then my life changed forever! I discovered Coach JC's program, and my first thought was, "it can't be this simple." He proved me wrong!

Coach JC's program changed my mindset, and it has revolutionized my outlook on what I eat and how I lose weight. I didn't realize how important eating right was

TRANSFORM YOUR THINKING

1

until he started coaching me. His philosophy was so different from what I had always heard, and I was just so glad that I didn't have to go on another diet.

Over the years I have wasted so much time in the gym. With Coach JC's program I am amazed at how much I can get done in such a short amount of time. The work-

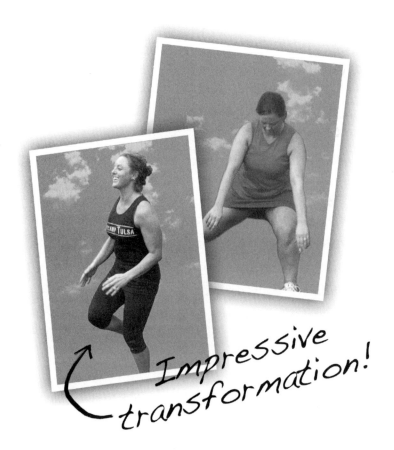

Impressive transformation!

outs are never easy, but with my busy schedule, I am able to maximize my time.

The best part: I am seeing the results that I have desired for so many years! To date, I have lost a total of 24 pounds, and I will continue to lose a few more. Many people have told me that it looks like I have lost more than 24 pounds, and that is because my body composition has also changed. My arms, legs, and butt are so much more toned, and everything on my body has firmed up.

I now look forward to working out and making myself a better person - a better person for myself and not for anybody else. My life has been transformed! I feel better and I look better, but most importantly, my health has improved so much during this time. I feel like I have been given the secret that I have been searching for all of these years.

Thank you, Coach JC, for all of your help, and thank you for investing these principals into my life. I am truly a changed person.

Jodi Hunt – 31 years old

CHAPTER EIGHT

DON'T FEAR FAILING

---

*Most of the things that I have accomplished in
life have been out of the fear of being mediocre.*

Fear can keep you from relationships, career opportunities,
losing weight, and ultimate happiness. A lot of people fear that
they are going to fail and that is why they never take the chance
to make it happen. Fear can paralyze you right where you are.
Fear is your worst enemy! What are you really afraid of? Are
you scared that you won't lose the weight that you desire? Are
you scared that you may put that weight right back on? This fear
can torture you if you don't take control of it now. This fear will
prevent you from achieving ultimate success. Think about how
many times in your past you knew that you could have done
something but did not act out of fear of failure. Really think
about it, what is the worst that could happen if you fail? You
learned the way not to do it and can now try again another way
to make it happen. A lot of people live in this fear, but if you
really think about it and what the outcome can be, it is never really that bad. If something doesn't work, it just did not work. So
what?! From here on out, you will be turning failure situations
into positive ones. Fear will become your partner, your friend.
From here on out, you will begin to take risks in life. Taking
risks in life is the only way to get ahead. The word risk may
scare you. I know what you are probably thinking, "If I take
risks, then there is going to be that chance of failure." Remember, you will now begin to not look at it as failure but as the way
not to do it.

You may be thinking or even saying, "I can't do that. I am
not a risk-taking person." Now, picture yourself 20 years from
now in the same physical state that you are currently in, picture
yourself at the same job in the same desk, and picture yourself

making the same amount of money. If you don't take any risks, this is what will happen. In 20 years, you will be exactly where you are today. You have to make the effort to change and go and take what you want. So the question is not, are you going to fail? Failure is going to happen, but from now on you are not going to look at it as failure. You are going to turn this into a positive, by figuring out what went wrong and applying what you learned so that next time you know what not to do. You cannot allow fear of failure to be part of your attitude. Your attitude cannot reflect fear. Instead, you will start to attack situations in life! You will take the necessary risks that will get you ahead in life! You will do this with your physical appearance, your relationships, your workplace, and with any other areas where you are not happy.

The biggest fear people face is the fear of failure. It is so powerful it can cripple your goals. This fear can keep you from accomplishing your dreams. It can even cause you to stop dreaming all together. I have seen this fear be so destructive that it has changed a person's entire course of life just so that he could avoid this fear of failure completely.

This fear will cause you to settle and to choose to live a mediocre life just so you can avoid certain situations. You cannot allow this fear to stunt your growth – the growth of your vision and the growth of your hope to have the body that you desire. This fear of failure may have been something that was inherited from family or friends or surroundings. This fear may not just show up sometimes but is constantly around; you may think about it on a daily basis. It may even haunt you and constantly remind you of why you haven't tried something. Maybe you wanted to try a new fitness program or try a new career but just never did it. This fear can really exert itself on you every moment of every day. I have seen a lot of people become a prisoner of this fear, unable to free themselves, unable to escape, simply because they allowed it to be that way. This fear may not cause you death, but it will rob you of living the life that you deserve to live, a life of enjoyment and fulfillment.

It's Time To Enjoy Life!

CHAPTER NINE

DECIDE TO LET GO OF THE PAST

You are who you are because of your past;
who will you be in the future?

Your past can haunt you and hold you back from accomplishing what you were called to do.

I have witnessed so many people that just could not let go of the past, and therefore, they let it control their future. Because of things that happened in the past, they were constantly dealing with feelings of depression, guilt, or anxiety. Some of them have even mentioned that to let go of the past would be impossible. First, let me say that nothing is impossible! Now is your time to let go of those things that have happened in the past.

You are probably thinking, "How can I let go of something that is so much a part of me?" I have been there, and I once questioned, "why let the past go?" The reason is simple, and it is this. If you live in the past, you will not be able to fully live in the present or in the future. You need to be who you are in the present! Yes, you may be who you are because of what happened to you in the past, but I want to tell you that you are more then that – you are in the present and you can only be who you are right now in the present. Who you are in the present will help determine your future!

A lot of people cling to the past in order to excuse themselves from being who they need to be in the present. Not you! At least not any more! It is time to face the reality of who you are now. The past is out of your control. Do not be controlled by something you cannot currently control. Starting today, you will not allow the past to determine who you are! You will not be bound and held down by feelings like anxiety, guilt, sadness, and depression. Letting go does not always mean forgetting the past.

These past memories, good or bad, are a part of us. The key is to realize that they are not the reality of who you are right now. The past will keep you stuck carrying extra baggage and weighing your life down. This garbage will hinder you from functioning at optimal performance. Now is the time to throw that garbage away, and now is the time to take those chains off for good. Free yourself forever!

I am here to tell you good news, and that is this: the now you can choose, the past is done, and the future is going to be awesome! That is, if you want it to be. I don't want you to hold yourself responsible for things that you cannot control, and you cannot control your past, so let it go. It is done! Now is the time to let go and move on so that you can have those things that you desire. Now is the time for you to have the body of which you always dreamed and the health that you deserve!

Now is the time for you to build the best body and the best life that you can imagine!

Check out what happened with Jennifer after she let the past go:

"I have tried it all to find the appropriate amount of calories to balance weight loss and being healthy for me. I have been at either extreme, going between not counting a single calorie that I ate, to eating 700-900 cals. a day and putting my body in starvation mode. I have wrecked havoc on my metabolism. I got married in May of 2007 and for the last year and a half have been trying desperately to lose weight. I tried running, a number of different gym classes, and even hired a personal trainer, I bought an elliptical machine and would work out for an hour a day at least 5 days a week. I finally sought the help of a nutritionist. Nothing that had worked for me in

TRANSFORM YOUR THINKING

1

the past was working, in fact I actually managed to gain 15 pounds in the process and I felt entirely out of control and helpless.

When I first heard about Coach JC's program I was not convinced that I would see the results that others were testifying to, but I figured I had nothing to lose. I joined the program 2 months ago and have lost 16 pounds so far. For a girl that has tried for over a year to even lose 2 pounds and seen no results, this was phenomenal

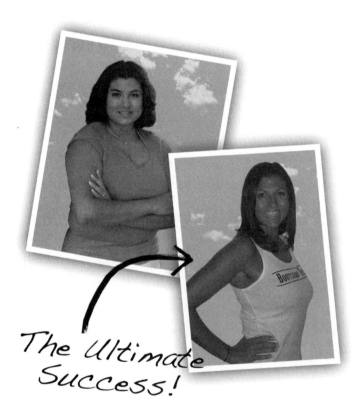

The Ultimate Success!

progress. I cannot believe the changes that I have experienced physically, mentally and emotionally. Coach JC is encouraging and truly cares! From Day 1 your health and fitness goals are made a priority and no matter your individual fitness level you are challenged each and every workout. It has helped me to become more confident, more outgoing and I finally feel back in control of my diet, fitness and overall health.

Coach JC's program is by far the most difficult workout I have ever been a part of, yet the results speak for themselves. I have more fun working out and I am in this for the long run. I plan to continue this program for many years to come... this is only the beginning."

Jennifer Lynn Frazier — 26 years old

TRANSFORM YOUR THINKING

CHAPTER TEN

DON'T EVER QUIT

Quitting is losing and losing is not winning!

The one type of person who has always bothered me is the quitter. I cannot stand to see someone just quit and give up! Still to this day, it angers me. This "quitter mentality" can really prevent you from accomplishing great things in life. If you have been a quitter in the past... not any more!

You need to establish a no–quit mentality. Tell yourself that you will never tap out. Sometimes people need to take other directions and maybe a different approach to ultimately see the results they desire. I am all for that. That is wisdom, to know what direction you need to take. I am talking about quitting; I am talking about giving up. Too many people quit too early. You see it every day in America. Look at the divorce rate. Look at all the unhappy people. Look at all the unhealthy ones. I really believe that people do not accomplish the things that they should simply because they quit and they quit too early. Consistency is the key in life. If you really want something to work, then you have to stick with it. So many people give up when things aren't going their way. You just don't know! Tomorrow could have been when the breakthrough came. Given another three weeks, and you may have broken that barrier and lost those extra ten pounds. You can't give up in life and you can't give up when you are trying to take control of your health. If you really want to get fit and have the body that you always wished, then you have to stick with the plan. Don't go searching for the newest diet pill or the next fad diet. Pick one that is proven to work and work it to the best of your ability. You have that plan right here in your hands, and I am telling you that if you do not give up, you will see the results that you want to see.

You Deserve Those Results... Don't Quit!

PART **2**

THE NEW YOU

CHAPTER ELEVEN

DO CHANGE YOUR THINKING

Change Your Thinking, Change Your RESULTS!

I once heard a preacher tell a story, and today I often share it with a lot of my clients. It was May 6, 1954, and no runner competing in track and field had ever run a mile in less than four minutes. All the so-called experts and commentators declared that it would never be done. Studies were performed to show that it was not humanly possible and that no one could possible run that fast for that long in order to make it happen. For years those tests and studies stood true and no one broke the four-minute mile barrier. However, on that day in 1954, a man named Roger Bannister made sports history and ran a mile in 3 minutes and 59 seconds! Up until that point, the runners allowed the opinions of others to dictate their outcome. Roger Bannister trained hard and did not believe what all the experts were saying. He did not believe that it was impossible. He refused to let others determine his outcome, and he believed that he would break that four-minute mile run. He did not allow others to put a limit on his life. He was going to determine his own future and his own destiny. This story is so fascinating not only because Roger Bannister made history, but also because of what I am about to tell you: just 46 days later, another runner broke his record. Now, after more than 50 years, hundreds of runners have run a mile in less than four minutes! I want you to think about that. For hundreds of years no one could run the mile in less than four minutes. It was pretty much accepted that no man could break the four-minute mile barrier. It was believed that the four-minute mile was physically impossible. It was commonly accepted as a fact! However, the reality was that the four-minute mile was a **psychological barrier!**

So what happened? I will tell you. For all those years athletes allowed others to set that barrier in their minds. For all those years runners believed what others said. Everyone was convinced that it was impossible. The lid was put on their lives. The power of the mind is incredible! These "limiting beliefs" or "mental barriers" are real and are a lot more powerful than people believe them to be.

I am here to tell you that you can't believe what others are saying: the media, your family members, magazines, other books, co-workers, etc. It is time to take the lid off of your life and start to break some records. It is time to think big! Change your thinking and you will change your results! It is time to believe that you can do it. It is time to remove all the fear and doubt from your life. Now is your time!

Now Is Your Time To Think Big!

CHAPTER TWELVE

DO THINK BIG

Beloved, I pray that in all respects you may prosper and be in good health, just as your soul prospers.

3 John 2

I train athletes on a regular basis, and a lot of the athletes that I deal with have big dreams. Dreams to be great at the sport they participate in, dreams to be the best in that sport. I am constantly telling them to dream big, and I want you to do the same. I tell these athletes that when you do everything that you know you need to do to prepare, then you should expect big things. What you expect from yourself is what you will get. Start to think big! Expect big things and big results! I don't accept an average work ethic from them, and I don't accept mediocre results. I demand that everything we do is in excellence! If we address it at this point, then it won't become a problem when competition is here. I want to challenge you today to expect big things! You must change your thinking before you can ever change your body. You do this by beginning to expect big things in your life. This is where it starts; later I will show you how to take this big thinking and begin to speak it until you see it. So many people settle in their mind for so little. I hear it all the time: "I got the best job I could with my education." "I lost all the weight that my genetics will allow me." "I can't make more money then I am now because I am at the highest position in the company." All of that is just a mindset, and that mindset is limiting your potential. It is time to take the limit off your life! Remove the lid! You can lose more weight! You can get a better job! Your marriage can be better! You can make more money! You can have the body that you have always wanted! Don't limit yourself by where you currently are or by what you currently have. Stop limiting yourself! I have found that people have so much more potential then they give themselves credit for. You have to believe in yourself. If you don't believe in yourself, why should anyone else?

I have seen people dream and believe much larger then I could ever imagine, much larger then anything visible that they had at the moment. You know what happened? They eventually stepped into what they believed they would be or what they believed they could have. From that point on, I started adopting the philosophy, "Fake It Until You Make It!" If you want to be healthy, start acting like you are healthy. If you want to be fit, how would you act if you were fit? If you want to change where you are in life, then start faking it until you make it. Start acting how you would act if you were already there. You know what is going to eventually happen? You will believe that you are that thing and then when you eventually are, you will just walk right into it and you will already know how to act.

Now let's be realistic: if you are a size 10 and you want to be a size 4, I am not telling you to try to fit into a size 4 every day and wear it around. That would be very uncomfortable and not such a pretty sight for everyone. What I am telling you is that now is your time to think bigger then you ever have. Don't limit yourself any longer!

Start to Fake It Until You Make It! Think as Big as You Possibly Can!

CHAPTER THIRTEEN

DISCOVER ACCOUNTABILITY

Accountability is making the decision to
allow others to make you great!

You will only go as far as you are accountable! It is amazing how so many people get uncomfortable when they hear the word accountability. Being accountable is a great thing and a must! So many people fail in life and in their fitness–related goals because they try to do it on their own. Life is not easy, so why try to attack it on your own? If you look at the people who are very successful in life, you will find that they had true accountability throughout the process. Times are going to be tough, the road is going to take a turn, and this is when that accountability will pull you through. You have to get accountable! This does not mean that I am telling you to trust everyone and anyone. What I am telling you is to find someone who you trust and respect, and allow them to make you better. This is someone who wants to see you achieve your goals and live your life to the fullest. This is someone who you can be totally open, honest, and vulnerable with at all times. In the beginning it may be a little uncomfortable, but once you get outside of your comfort zone, you will be able to confront and address those difficult issues and weaknesses in your life.

Accountability is simple and this is how it works. You will inform this person whom you trust of your goals and what you are trying to accomplish. Then you will inform them of what you believe is going to be the most difficult part of the process for you. You will ask them to help keep you motivated and not to let you quit or get off track. You will ask them to hold you accountable to your weaknesses, such as late–night snacking. You will ask them to call you in the evening to check up and remind you that you don't need a snack and to remind you why you are doing what you are doing. I have found that it works really well if you can find an accountability partner that is reaching for the same goals as you – this way you can hold each other accountable and go through the process together. You know the saying that iron sharpens iron! Encouragement and moral support from a friend are sometimes the missing ingredients in fighting the battle against weight loss and getting fit.

Get accountable today and get fit for life!

30 pounds, 29 inches, and 10 percent body fat!

"Before I met Coach JC and his team, I had decided that I wanted to change my life around. I was very overweight

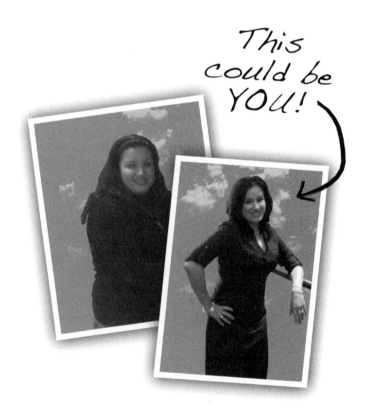

and unhappy about it. I was working out at the gym everyday but not getting the results I wanted. It took me four months to drop seven pounds, which I gained back by Christmas. In January 2009, I made a life-changing decision, I joined Coach JC's program. It is more than just a workout; this program has given me the encouragement, accountability, and knowledge needed to transform my life! I am a healthy person and I don't have to worry about gaining my weight back. It has taught me to make better choices, and I am able to do exercises I never thought I could do. Thanks to Coach JC, I have lost 30 pounds, 29 inches, and 10 percent body fat (and this is just my fourth month!)."

Miriam Tover — 28 years old

CHAPTER FOURTEEN

DEVELOP A SENSE OF URGENCY

Without a sense of urgency, desire loses its value.

Jim Rohn

Now Is Your Time!

Do you have a sense of urgency? How badly do you want to lose that weight? How badly do you want to take control of your health? It is time to get out of your comfort zone and get back in the race! Do me a favor and start to observe successful people. Have you noticed that people who make things happen in life are those that posses a sense of urgency? A sense of urgency is something that successful people possess. A sense of urgency is established when something is of great importance to you, it is a necessity. You need to have it or do it. A lot of times this sense of urgency can bring some pressure. A pressure to demand yourself that it gets done. Starting today, you need to feel that accomplishing your goal is a matter of life and death. I believe that a lot of times, true greatness is birthed from a sense of urgency. You cannot afford to prolong your dreams and goals any longer. You owe it to yourself and your loved ones to be healthy and live a life of longevity. Are you willing to pay the price? Are you willing to do whatever it takes? We all want to have a great body and live free of diseases, but the question is, are you willing to put the time in to do whatever it takes to accomplish your dreams and goals? You have to do it! It is now or never! You know that if you don't take control of it now, it is only going to get worse. This is where a sense of urgency comes into play. You must have the attitude that you would rather be dead then live a mediocre life. It is now or never!

That is why I have made this a coaching program, a game plan, to give you time limits. Time limits will help you establish that sense of urgency. Think about it for a second: all the things that affect you on a daily basis, if there was no deadline, no sense of urgency, how would your daily life be different? Time limits are crucial. With newspapers that are printed each day, each department has deadlines so that it can be edited and printed. Stoplights are on a timer to ensure that traffic travels smoothly. Planes, trains, buses, and subways all use schedules to create a sense of action from their customers. Most of your appointments are scheduled and depend on a sense of urgency. Life is one big time limit! These time limits are used simply to give people a sense of responsibility and accountability and to ensure that things get completed efficiently. Take action today and stay focused on the task at hand. Realize what is at the end of the tunnel.

How badly do you really want it? How urgent is it to you?

THE NEW YOU

2

CHAPTER FIFTEEN

DO GET BACK IN THE RACE

For a race to be finished, you must first start.

Ask any runner and they will tell you that it is not about how you start but how you finish. That is true, but how will you ever finish if you do not start? If things don't start right you can't give up, you have got to keep running. Maybe you have tried to get fit before, maybe you have tried diet after diet, maybe you have even hired a personal trainer, but you weren't seeing the results, so you dropped out of the race. Today, I want you to get back into the race. Maybe this book is the starting point for your race. To finish the race, you first have got to start the race. I don't care what happened in the past, your new race begins today. Today is the day you get back into the race – the race of life. Think of every day of your life as just one lap in the competition of your race. Once that lap is over you will never get it back, and once the race is over, it's over. Life is short and once it is over it is over. There is not another race. The race of life is to complete what you know you were called to do. I am not just talking about getting back into the race but finishing the race strong. Today, I want you to re-submit your name, put your sneakers on, and get back into the race. Once you get back in, then you will have a chance to win the race. The race for everyone is going to be different. In this race, you are racing against yourself. You have to win this one for yourself, but also for your loved ones and the people that need you. What about your kids, your family, other people that need you? Remember, you getting your health back is going to help a lot of people get their health back too.

There will always be someone trying to take you back out of the race, and in the past, you may have allowed this to occur. Not any longer! When someone or a circumstance threatens to take you out and steal your joy of accomplishing that goal, you will not allow it to happen. You must refuse to be knocked down; you must refuse to be knocked out. You are to keep running and not look back. If you need a drink, don't even stop, grab one as you keep going. Nothing slows you down and nothing ever again will take you back out of the race. Starting today, you will start strong and you will finish strong!

Now let me show you what can happen when you decide to get back into the race, allow accountability to work in your life and make the decision that you will never quit:

20 Pounds and Size 14 to Size 10!

"The results I've seen have been exactly what I hoped would happen while training with Coach JC. I have lost 20 pounds and have dropped from a size 14 to a 10. My waist, thighs, and backside are much smaller. Coach JC's coaching style is nothing but outstanding! He is the most motivated man I have met and his disposition is always positive and encouraging. He wants every woman who works out with him to be successful. Coach JC always gives his clients positive feedback and encourages them to be the best they can be. Coach JC has a wealth of information about exercise, nutrition, and how to get you to meet your exercise goals. It doesn't matter if you are a professional athlete or a mom who just wants to be in better shape, he will motivate you and help you attain your full potential. My life before his program was pretty busy with work, my family, and trying to keep up with laundry and a clean house. I didn't give myself any time during the day for myself and I was starting to feel "old." After training with Coach JC's program I started to feel

THE NEW YOU

2

more energetic; I was sleeping better, and I had one hour of time just for me. Now that I have been in the program for months, I would say that I am addicted to it. If I miss a workout I have such guilt and can't wait until the next one. My life is still busy with work, my family, and trying to keep up with laundry and a clean house, but I have made time for me and that's the most important thing. I am a better wife and mother since I have a place to work off some of the stress and worries of the day. I am stronger both physically and mentally, my flexibility is great, and my body is almost where I want it to be. Coach JC's program has been the best workout to help me achieve my goal of a healthier lifestyle. This is what Coach JC's program has done for me!"

Mindy Fleming — 43 years old

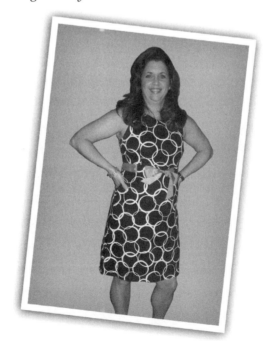

CHAPTER SIXTEEN

DO EXPECT RESULTS

If you don't believe in yourself, why should anyone else believe in you?

Expect Results! Preparation time is never wasted time. If you do what you need to do, then you should expect results. I always tell my athletes: the ones who are disciplined and who put the time into training and preparing should expect good things. They should expect results. Once you start to implement the program and implement it to the fullest, then you should expect to see the results you desire. The mind is a powerful weapon. If you don't believe in yourself, then why should anyone else believe in you? I am not talking about being cocky and arrogant. I am talking about confidence, a confidence that you are taking care of business, that you are back into the race, and that you are not going to quit until you reach your final goal. The only one that can take you out of the game is yourself. While you are on the field you can't be defeated, while you are on the court you can't lose, while you are in the race you are the best on the track. Remember the only one that can take you out of the race is you! Start expecting results, start expecting good things, and start expecting your life to take a turn in the right direction! You can now have a peace of mind to know that you have the right program. The time of doubting yourself is over! Expect great things in your life, and expect that you will see the results you desire. Have confidence that you can do it and you will lose the weight and get fit. Expect results knowing that you are doing what is right. Expect results now that you are taking the risks needed to take control of your life. You now have the knowledge that you need to do it. You have committed to finish the race and you are focused. Now is time to expect results; never doubt that you can do it!

I believe in you! Believe in yourself!

CHAPTER SEVENTEEN

DO KNOW THAT
WHAT YOU SOW YOU SHALL REAP

"Be not be deceived; God is not mocked:
for whatsoever a man soweth, that shall he also reap."

Galatians 6:7

You have probably heard this said before and I have found it to be very true in many different aspects of life. "What you sow, you will reap." If you sow badly you will reap badly; if you sow well you will reap well. If all you eat is junk food, you will reap the negative rewards of the junk food. The saying, "you are what you eat" is actually very true. No, I don't think you will actually turn into that food, but it will definitely be reflected in your physique. You have to start sowing well – in what you eat, in your lifestyle, and in your fitness. As you start to follow the game plan, you will reap the benefits of eating well. As you follow the game plan, you will see those pounds fall off. Be enthusiastic as you do what you must do to conquer your health. I see so many people who are getting into shape looking miserable. First off, it is because their workout routine is boring and dull. You should enjoy taking control of your health, and you will with this 27-day transformation program. You should be enthusiastic about your future. Every day you are going to be one step closer to your ultimate goal; every day you will be conquering something in your life. Be excited about the body you are going to have, be excited about increasing your productivity in all that you, be excited about being alive and having the opportunity to live life to the fullest. Don't be afraid to have some enthusiasm about what you are doing because this will become contagious. You will start to see other areas of your life improving. Remember, you have a fabulous future to look forward to and you should enjoy life today and every step along the way.

I started working with Coach JC after losing about 50 lbs, needing to lose more weight but was completely stuck. He provided a clear, easy-to-follow game plan to change my eating habits and increase the intensity of my workouts. I went for it full-force and have achieved results far beyond what I expected - I'm in the best shape of my life and am down three sizes! I'm even training for a 15K race - something I never thought I'd attempt before working with Coach JC. Just beware of one side effect...clothes-shopping is a whole lot more fun when you're constantly looking for smaller sizes!

As you're going through this process, just remember that transforming your health and fitness is an investment in yourself - in your future. It takes work and consistency - and is worth every effort!

Deborah Wipf – 28 years old

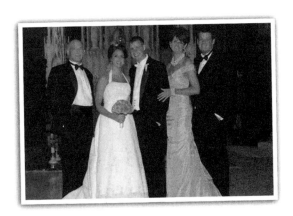

THE NEW YOU

2

CHAPTER EIGHTEEN

DO BE A CONTROL FREAK

First we make our habits, then our habits make us.

Charles C. Noble

Your future is in your hands. You control your future, and you determine what happens tomorrow. This is your life, so control the outcome of it. I talk to so many people who have allowed other people and other people's situations to determine where they are currently. I once was speaking to an ex-convict who had been in prison for four years. I sat there why he told me his story and to sum it up, he was locked away because someone set up a robbery, and he drove the vehicle to the robbery. Things did not go well. Four guys were convicted, and he was one of them. All he did was drive the car. One guy was the mastermind who set everything up and arranged the robbery and four guys went down. This guy was in prison for four years, and still he did not want to take responsibility for the actions that send him to prison. No one forced him to do what he did. He was in complete control of his life, and he allowed one little instant to change his life forever.

So many people let their bodies get so out of shape and don't want to take control of the outcome. No one made you eat Mc-Donald's every day. I can hear you making the excuse now, "But it was on the way to work." No one made the decision for you to not be active, to not exercise, and to let your body go downhill. You are at this point in your life today because of the choices that you made yesterday. You control your future, and you control your health. Be a control freak. It is your life! Take control of it!

Your desire to be fit, to lose weight, and to conquer that area of your life must be strong; it must be strong enough to overcome mental laziness. Everyone wants the easy way out. Do not allow that mental laziness to determine your future. I won't let you do it. Not any more! You are going to work to get the results, but you are going to work wise so that these results, once achieved, begin to work for you. They will work for you as long as you want them to, as long as you allow them to.

Start to become a control freak and control your future from now on!

THE NEW YOU

2

PART 3

TIME TO GET MOVING

CHAPTER NINETEEN

DO TAKE ACTION

I don't know the key to success, but the key to
failure is trying to please everyone.

Bill Cosby

You have to get started. You have to start making some forward progress. You have to get a little momentum. Have you ever heard the saying, "Those who do not suffer defeats are those who are not in the fights?" If you are not fighting to accomplish your goals then you will never get defeated, but you will also never reach your goals. A lot of people never get to where they need to simply because they never get started. You have to get started! Most people don't get started because of that fear issue we spoke about earlier. We already addressed that, and it is not a problem any longer. Let's get the ball rolling. You have the desire for change in your life, you have no more excuses, you are not afraid any longer, your attitude is in check, your priorities are set, you know what you are after, and you have set the goals to get there... Now Get Moving! Don't procrastinate any longer. I don't care what your plans are for today. Today is the day you gain momentum; today is the day you start moving one step closer to your ultimate goal. When you are finished reading this chapter, I want you to put the book down and do something that is going to benefit you and get you started on the path to that ultimate goal. Maybe it is doing some jumping jacks or maybe it is going to the kitchen to clean the junk food out of the pantry. Whatever it is, today it needs to start. It takes at least 21 to 30 days to develop a habit. My goal for you is to develop a habit, a lifestyle change, in your 27-day game plan. Once the habit is established, it becomes part of your everyday activity and it becomes a lot easier. If you don't get started, you will never reach the 27th day. Movement is a requirement for a goal-orientated person. Nothing happens for those who just sit and wish. You can wish all day that you were back to a size eight. You can dream all day about being a millionaire, but without action, all it will ever be is a dream. When you are not moving forward, you are moving backwards. There is no just remaining the same; there is no just standing still. Think about it, water that is not moving becomes stagnant very quickly. Over time, that water becomes nasty and moldy. It doesn't stay clear, clean water. It regresses, just like the human body. Once again, this is where no risk, no reward comes into play. To get moving you may have to become a little uncomfortable. You may have to get out of that comfort zone, but remember, do you really want to be exactly where you are today in 20 years? Remember, the worst feeling in the world is the feeling of regret – to have to look back and ask yourself the question what if or if only?

Movement creates momentum; creation is who you are and what you do. You create your present and you create your future! Start to create your future by taking action today. Once you get moving, keep moving, and remember don't ever quit.

Check out Donna who didn't quit until she saw that which she desired. Once she started moving, she could not be stopped!

"JC and his training are the real deal! He is passionate and has combined his God-given talents with hard work, discipline, and consistency. He expects nothing out of anyone else that he hasn't done or will do – right along side of you. He is serious about your overall health and well-being. He works to get you out of your comfort zone and into living a healthy, more active lifestyle.

While utilizing Coach JC's program for over three months, I lost 15 pounds and 7.9 percent body fat, which included the following body measurement reductions:

Thigh: 2.5 inches

Hips: 2 inches

Waist: 2 inches

Chest: 1.5 inches

Cholesterol: 33 Point Drop

Before joining this program, I was a "fluffy mother" who had just about decided to welcome my new body type and learn to love it. I have never had a weight problem and have been a busy wife, mother, business owner, and volunteer, to name a few things. I was constantly at meetings, on and off airplanes, sitting at my computer, driving here and there – always on the move. Then, over the last year, I gained over 20 pounds. For the first time, it was uncomfortable for me to tie my shoe and it seemed like my clothes needed an update. I found myself complaining about not enough close parking, sitting whenever I could, and looking for looser fitting styles of clothing. After I had my annual physical and found out that there was nothing wrong with me, I was ready to accept life's wrinkles and bumps and to join the new elderly.

Since completing the program, I have continued a modified, healthier lifestyle. I have lost an additional six pounds and my cholesterol has dropped another thirty points over the year following the program. I look for opportunities instead of excuses for good exercise. Now, my whole family trains with Coach JC. My younger son will

TIME TO GET MOVING

3

be ready to play college football and my older son will be physically fit and ready as he works to get on with the fire department. My husband's increased energy, strength, and lower blood pressure have been a tremendous qual-ity-of-life gift. We have all worked so hard at this point, and none of us would ever want to go back to how we felt before Coach JC!"

Donna Weinkauf — 48 years old

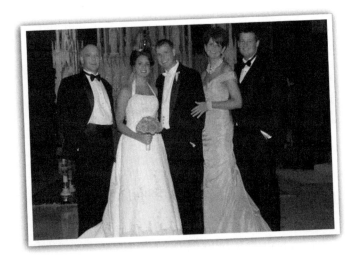

CHAPTER TWENTY

DO BECOME AGILE

Don't let obstacles stop you. If you run into a wall,
don't turn around and give up, figure out how to
climb it, go through it, or work your way around it.

Agility is simply defined as the ability to get from point A to point B in the shortest amount of time, while losing the least amount of motion. Listen, obstacles are going to occur, times are going to get tough, the road will be rocky, and that is a guarantee. The question is, what are you going to do when these inevitable circumstances occur? Starting today, you need to become agile. Being agile is a huge component of being a great athlete. We train our athletes to become more agile so that they can perform at the highest level. For you to be successful and to accomplish what you desire, you will need to become both agile in the physical and in the mental. When your mind becomes agile, you will be able to conquer anything. Watch how quickly the pounds fall off! What are you going to do when obstacles come at you? When these obstacles come at you, you have to do whatever it takes to not let them stop you. Nothing can stop you! I don't care if you have to go through, around, over, or under. Whatever you have to do you must do it. This is something that is developed; increasing your agility can be trained just like it can physically in an athlete. You must make a conscious effort on a daily basis to fight through obstacles. When tough times come at you, go around them. Every day a situation will arise that will make you uncomfortable, so practice becoming more agile. Use daily circumstances to make yourself better so that when the large obstacles are thrown at you, you will know how to react.

It's time to become agile!

CHAPTER TWENTY ONE

DETERMINE YOUR PRIORITIES

*You can always tell what someone really wants
in life by looking at their priorities.*

What are your priorities? Do you know why a lot of people are overweight and don't have control of their health? It is because losing weight is not a priority! What is it that you really value in life? You can always tell a person's desires and values by their priorities. What are your priorities?

Now is the time to address the priorities in your life! Most people generally understand the meaning of priority, but few people prioritize their life and activities on a daily basis. I speak with people all the time about their priorities, and it always amazes me to see the difference between what they say and what their actions really reflect. Your priorities are not expressed by what you say, but rather by your daily actions. You may know in your heart that you want to lose weight and live a healthy lifestyle, but it is the follow through, the action that is slowing down your progress.

I want to give you five steps to prioritize your priorities:

1. Know what you want and don't waiver from it.

2. Write it out – Make it clear and be specific and realistic.

3. Live it out – Walk it out on a daily basis. Be who you say you are!

4. Associate Yourself – Surround yourself with people that have like priorities.

5. Give it a checkup – Re-evaluate your priority list on a weekly or monthly basis.

Now, stop talking about it. Go and run with it!

CHAPTER TWENTY TWO

DISCOVER GOAL SETTING

*Setting goals is the first step in turning
the invisible into the visible."*

Anthony Robbins

If you don't know what you want, you will never get it. If you don't know where you are going, you will never get there. Setting goals will help lead you to where you want to go in life. Knowing where you want to go enables you to concentrate your activities and actions and efforts on the things that are necessary. A lot of the successful people who I admire have not only set goals, but have chased those goals until they reached them.

I am never amazed when I sit down with a client and I ask them, "What are your goals?" They may say to play in the NBA, to lose 35 pounds, or to pack on 25 pounds of muscle. Most people don't even need to think about it. A lot of people have determined their ultimate long-term goal, and that is great. I then follow up by asking them, "What are you doing to get there?" Very few people set short-term goals. What do you need to do on a daily basis? What about on a weekly basis? Or even a monthly and annual basis to get to this ultimate goal? Goal setting is crucial, but without the game plan to get you there, you will never see those goals come to pass. In the next 27 days you are going to set goals and have fun doing it. The great thing is that I am providing you with the game plan right here in this book to be successful and reach those goals.

Check this out! All you have to do is just do it.

Hiding behind scrubs, refusing to wear jeans, and several break downs inside countless dressing rooms was who I had become. I had convinced myself that black stretch pants and a black sweater made my size 16 frame look small. Huge misconception ladies and gentleman, look at my before picture, black is not slimming!

I have struggled with my weight my entire life. I can name you diets from A to Z that include eating all of one food, eating nothing but green, and even ones that included hardly eating at all. Beyond dieting, I am well versed in elliptical machines, treadmills, and the insides

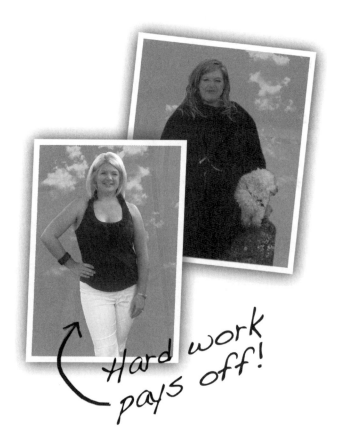

Hard work pays off!

of gyms. I even hired a personal trainer before my wedding to help me get fit for my big day.

After my wedding day the 12 pounds I had managed to lose creped back with a vengeance. Within one month, I had packed over half those pounds back on. And 4 months later every pound and a few more had made a home along my midsection and my hips. I had clearly reached the title of married, fat, and happy! I had passed wedding bliss, collected my extra baggage and I was settling in at 210 pounds.

"You'd be perfect for this!" These were the words that Coach JC said to me the day I met him at a local trade show. Me and my extra fluffiness, perfect for boot camp? I was more than hesitant, but he gave me a free pass and told me to give it a try. I convinced my best friend to give it a try with me and in February with the help of Coach JC my life changed.

I remember my first boot camp with Coach JC, although I could barely finish the exercises, Coach JC was there every step to encourage me and push me to that next level. Coach JC lit a fire in me and I couldn't wait to get to my next work out. In my first month of working with Coach JC I had lost 10 pounds! That wasn't my greatest success though, I was feeling great, I had more

TIME TO GET MOVING

3

strength, more confidence, and I was finding happiness
with myself again.

Not only has Coach JC been a constant motivator
in my body transformation, but he has evaluated and
modified my diet so that I can achieve optimum success.
These modifications and the tools Coach JC has given me
changed my eating habits. My body is a temple and putting junk and garbage in it is worthless and empty. I have
just completed my sixth month under Coach JC, and the
fire is burning bright! Coach JC has helped me to lose 38
pounds! Not only have I lost 38 pounds, but last month
at my cousin's wedding, I wore a size 8 dress. I saw family that I had not seen since my wedding, and I had to
pick their jaws up off the floor. My confidence was radi-
ating, and I owe it to Coach JC.

Coach JC has instilled in me good eating habits and he
has transformed my workouts. But, it is my increased
levels of confidence and happiness that has transformed
the most. Coach JC helped me to realize that I am worth
it, my body is worth it, and I can make the changes necessary to live a life of greater health and happiness. As
you can see, with Coach JC, I made the changes and look
at me now! Remember, you are worth it and your body is
worth it!

Taylor Deatherage - 26 years old

CHAPTER TWENTY THREE

DECIDE TO SPEAK IT

Begin to speak those things that you desire and want to accomplish. Let me start by saying that I don't believe you can just repeatedly say that you want something and it will happen. I am talking about speaking with a confidence and a positive attitude, while at the same time believing without a doubt that those things that you are working at will work out. If you repeatedly say, "I am going to lose those 20 pounds!" Then you will subconsciously find ways to make yourself lose those 20 pounds. You will start to believe that it is already a reality; therefore, you do what's necessary to make it happen. You must understand that this can work in a negative way also. If you keep saying, "I'll never lose these 20 pounds," you won't make any effort, and you will eventually quit because your subconscious mind will have accepted that you will never lose the weight. The other reason I believe that this is so powerful is that you will have people who will speak against you accomplishing your goal, people who do not want you to succeed, and people who will doubt that you can do it. The way to counteract this negativity is for you to defeat them by speaking against them. When you speak against this negativity, you are releasing your confidence, and you are exposing yourself to positive energy. You will never really experience true success in your life if you are negative and are always speaking depressing and doubtful things. When you constantly speak negatively, it can make you unpleasant to be around and very unhappy.

Don't get me wrong; I don't believe that everything you say will miraculously happen. People speak things they want all the time, but if you don't put action behind it, it's very rarely going to materialize. I am a big action guy! Here is the cool thing, speaking your goal into existence can considerably improve your results and how you feel about yourself and others. We all know these kinds of people! This is just very basic human nature. People who are happy and positive like to be around happy and positive people.

It goes back to what you sow is what you will reap. If you speak positively, you will get that back and positive things tend to happen. Now, why is this so powerful for you? It is because you are not only speaking it, but you are putting action behind it. That is what the game plan is all about, and that is a powerful combination! It always makes me laugh when someone says that there is no power in words. Chances are good that if someone said something hurtful to you as a kid, you have probably have never forgotten it! In fact, it may even still bother you. Maybe someone told you that you couldn't do something, and then you started to think that maybe you couldn't, and it stopped you from accomplishing something in your life. On the flip side, has anyone ever said something so positive to you that it encouraged you to take a step in your life that you were afraid to take? I know that this has happened to me.

So, let me be the first to start to speak into your life. I want to tell you that I believe in you, and I believe that you will accomplish your goal. I don't care if it is 10 pounds or 250 pounds, I believe that you can do it, and I believe that you will not quit until you get there. I have faith in you and I know that you will execute your dreams. I wrote this book because I want to help you fulfill those dreams and help you live your life to the fullest!

Now I want for you to hear from one of my clients that has made this program a priority in her life:

"Coach JC's Program has completely changed the way
I look at working out! I LOVE to work out now; yes
even at 5:30 AM! I used to dread going to the gym; and
found any excuse to not make it most days. But with
this program the work-outs are fun! You're not doing the
same old running on a treadmill and pointless crunches.

Coach JC is very motivating and makes sure everyone is getting the BEST workout for their exercise level.

This program has completely changed the way I look and feel about ME! I have more energy throughout the day, and I have started eating much smarter (you don't want to do all that hard work and throw it away on fast food)! At the end of the day, I just plain feel better; both physically and emotionally!!!

Thanks Coach JC!!! This program not only helped me achieve workout goals, but it has changed my outlook on living a better, healthier life!!"

Tasha Gabriel — 28 years old

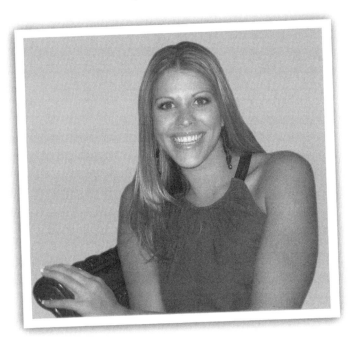

TIME TO GET MOVING

3

CHAPTER TWENTY FOUR

DO REALIZE IT IS A CHOICE

How badly do you really want it? How badly do you really want to be in shape? How badly do you really want to live a ful-filled life? How badly do you really want to lose that weight? Well, I have great news for you. Now you can go and live that great, fulfilled life! Now you can go and get into the best shape of your life! Now is your time. You may be saying to yourself, "It is just not that simple." Of course it is. All it takes is a choice. Just one decision – made by you! This may be something that you have always known, but today, I want you to allow it to become a revelation to you. I want you to allow it to become real. As you probably realize, much of life is a routine, and I have seen a lot of people become stale and stagnant. If you are not careful, it is very easy to fall into this trap. Make a decision starting to-day that you are not going to live another day on cruise control. Make a decision today that you are not going to allow your life to become stagnant. Have some passion about who you are, and make the decision to be passionate about what you are doing. It is your choice! Yes, it is that simple. So many people allow others to make decisions for them on a daily basis; they allow people to choose their future for them. Not me, and not you! You may not have the perfect body, you may not have the perfect job, you may not live in the perfect environment, but remember, you can still choose to change any of that. It is just a choice, just one decision! Today, you are choosing to take control of your life by taking control of your HEALTH. Today, you are choosing to take control of your health by taking control of your THINKING. You choose your future. You choose what your body looks like. You choose how much money you make. You choose what religion you practice. It's your choice. You choose who you are. That's great news!

If you ever want to be successful at anything in life, then you have to make the decision to want to make your life better. There are too many indecisive people in the world today and because of this, they never get anything accomplished. Their reply to everything is, "Let me think about it." Listen, you are done thinking about it. Starting today, I want you to make a decision. Make the decision that your life is valuable and that you are worth it. You are done thinking about it! Starting today, you will no longer make excuses and you will no longer accept anything else but greatness, you will no longer accept anything else but results! For me personally, whenever I make a tough decision, things just start to happen. You must make a decision to create an opportunity in your life that you may not have had otherwise.

TIME TO GET MOVING

3

CHAPTER TWENTY FIVE

DO BELIEVE IN YOURSELF

On a daily basis, I talk to many people who just don't believe that they can do it. You have to believe in YOU! As we go through life, we face different situations and problems that make us doubt ourselves. Sometimes we get really down and out, and things just don't go our way. I want to tell you that you are a winner! The past is the past. You have been made with a purpose, and you can do this! You have to be optimistic about yourself, you have to believe in your dreams, and you have to believe that you are going to achieve those things. You have to believe that you are going to lose that desired weight because you have changed your thinking and have the game plan. Believe that now is your time, and believe that this is the body that you deserve. Shoot, if you don't believe in you, why should anyone else?

You are valuable and you were born for a purpose! So many people just go through life and never accomplish their goals and what they were called to do on this earth. I don't care what you have been told and I don't care what you currently believe.The value system in our society has created people to put a lid on their life. Society may have even put a limit on your self worth, but not any longer. I don't care what your education is and I don't care what kind of car you drive. These are not the things that determine your self worth. Today I want for you to stop comparing yourself to everyone and everything else and I want for you to become the person that you know you were destined to become. It is your time for breakthrough! Your life has a purpose and you are valuable and it is time for you to experience your life for what it should be.Life is too short and to valuable to not believe in yourself...

CHAPTER TWENTY SIX

DO JUST DO IT

Now it is your time! You have learned over the last few chapters how to take control of your life. This chapter will be short and sweet. You are about to get all of the tools that you will need. Now is where the action comes into play. I would be foolish to tell you that these next 27 days will be easy, but I can tell you that it is simple. It is simple if you just do it! Commit to not just doing it but to do it the best you possibly can. So many people do things half heartily. I am telling you that what you put into these next 27 days is what you will get. It goes back to, How bad do you really want this? You have been given an opportunity; an opportunity to transform your body and transform your life forever. An opportunity to start over so that you can have the body that you desire and live the life of longevity that you deserve. What are you going to do with this opportunity? I have a great idea...Give it everything that you got and see what happens. I want you to really think about this...In just 27 days your life can be different! In just 27 days you could be on your way to ultimate success! In just 27 days you can have the body that you always desired! Can you go as hard as you can go for 27 days? Can you give it everything that you got? Can you not just do it but do it like there is no tomorrow. Is your life worth 27 days? Actions speak louder than words: Show me what you got! Just Do It!!!

TIME TO GET MOVING

3

CHAPTER TWENTY SEVEN

THE GAME PLAN

When it comes to exercise and nutrition, so many opinions exist that it may seem overwhelming. However, this game plan will clear through the clutter and confusion and provide you with mindset clarity, an effective workout routine and real life nutrition coaching advice. I have made this game plan simple, effective, and fun so that you can easily fit it into this festival that is better known as life.

For the next 27 days you will have the plan of action to succeed. I have given you a step-by-step, day-by-day game plan for you to lose the weight that you have always desired, to get fit, and to have the body of your dreams. I am giving you the tools necessary to be successful. What you do with those tools is up to you. You must execute every day for each of the 27 days to produce great results. You should strive to master the keys to success for each day to see the most optimal results.

Each day you will be given three transformation keys to be successful:

1. **The Secret To Real Weight Loss Success!**

2. **Transform Your Eating!**

3. **Transform Your Body!**

In the ***The Secret To Real Weight Loss Success*** section I will give you the step-by-step approach to conquer your thinking. In the first 26 chapters of this book, I addressed each one of these keys. Now for the next 27 days you will be given a systematic game plan on how to master those keys so that you can live the best life yet. This is where true success happens! Remember, you must change your mind before you can change your body!

In the *Transform Your Eating* section you will be given nutrition key each day to help you successfully lose the weight that you desire and to live a healthy life. Remember, this is not a diet. This is a lifestyle change. I am going to give you real life keys to eating so that you can experience ultimate health and weight loss. I want to show you how having the proper nutrition is not as difficult as people make it.

Remember, this is a coaching program. These are nutritional coaching suggestions. Are you coachable? In your game plan, I will be introducing you to a nutrition program that works! This program will help you improve your health, the way you look, and the way you feel. Some of these concepts may be new to you, but please know that we have been using this system for several years now. It has effectively helped hundreds of people to look better, feel better, and perform better.

Let me state once again that this is not another diet book! You will not count calories, and you will not just eat lettuce while starving yourself for months and hating life! Like I have mentioned numerous times, it takes hard work and discipline to accomplish your goals. These 27 days are no different. These 27 days are about change! I will coach you on how to feed your body so that you can achieve your health-related and weight-loss goals. I speak to people all the time who have a whole bookshelf filled with diet books, which poses my second question: with all of the information out there, why are we classified as an obese country? Why is child obesity on the rise? Why are people dying every day from health-related diseases?

Look at all the information out there and all the diet books. How many diet books have you purchased? Where are they now? Now, let me ask you a question, did they work for you?

Diets are a quick fix that promise you amazing and quick results. When you want to lose weight, is your first choice to find the latest fad diet or diet pill? Well, not any more! In the begin-

TIME TO GET MOVING

3

ning of a diet, a quick five to ten pounds might come off, but what happens when you return to your old eating habits? You find yourself back at the same weight or more within a few months. So, do diets work? On most diets, you are not eating the way you like to eat or the way you will eat for the rest of your life. You eat foods you may not even like and don't find satisfying. Some determined people might stick with the diet until they reach their goal, but here is the problem: you know you are determined and you do it "just for the diet." In this game plan, I will show you that there is an easier way you lose weight. Rather than chasing the next diet or fat-loss pill, I will help you find healthier foods you enjoy, in amounts that will not cause weight gain. Now, let me tell you some other reasons why we don't use diets with our clients.

THE WORD "DIET" IS NO FUN!

We have found that the very word "diet" is depressing to most people. You hear "diet," and you FREAK OUT! You think of giving up foods that are enjoyable to you. Okay, who wants to get together with friends at a party and munch on celery sticks while others are eating cheesecake? We have even seen some people stop socializing because of their dieting. In America, food has become a big part of how we interact with our friends and family. When you feel deprived of what you enjoy and even alienated from people who are not dieting, you will eventually quit. Then (and this is the big problem) you will go back to the way you were eating – the way that wasn't working in the first place!

DON'T BE A YO-YO!

Yo-yo dieting can be dangerous and detrimental to a person's health. There are some dangers associated with the yo-yo diet cycle of losing weight, gaining it back, losing it again, gaining it back, and then maybe even gaining more then when you started! It can be stressful on your body's organs to have fluctuating swings in body weight. Additionally, diets actually slow down your metabolism! To lose weight you need to exercise and eat right. Your game plan will give you the knowledge on how to do this.

In the ***Transform Your Body*** section I will be introducing you to my famous Bootcamp Tulsa workout. This is the same workout that has produced some unbelievable results in people all over the world. This is the same workout routine that helped famous musician, Tom Basler, to lose 104 pounds in just fifteen weeks. This is the same workout that has transformed many people's lives so they can live life to the fullest once again. Before we get started, I want you to hear from one of those people. I hope YOU are one of my next testimonials!

Famous Musician Loses 104 Pounds and is still going!

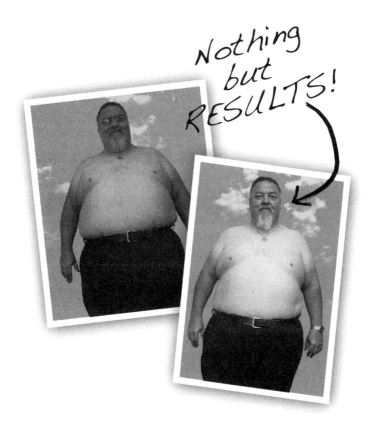

TIME TO GET MOVING

3

"I started training with Coach JC in January 2009 when I weighed over 500 pounds. My family doctor had told me three months prior that he didn't expect me to live ten years without dramatic weight loss and lifestyle changes. I was also being treated for ulcer-like wounds on my shins that weren't healing; the Wound Specialist informed me I was a good candidate for amputation. I was placed in the pre-screening stages for Gastric Bypass surgery. I really didn't want to have the surgery but couldn't think of alternatives. Dieting had never given me any long-term results; in fact, I believe "dieting" got me into the situation I was in. I was introduced to Coach JC and the work began. It was a pretty serious project since my mobility and capacity to exercise was severely limited. Initially, we couldn't even find a scale capable of weighing me. The nutrition program started before the exercise because I had to be cleared by my family doctor. On January 14, I did my first workout. It wasn't much, and it hurt, but I had started. We arbitrarily guessed my starting weight at 500 pounds; though it could have been as much as 530 to 550 pounds. The first actual weight we recorded was 467 pounds. I am now at 396 pounds and have been consistently losing five and a half to seven pounds per week. I know this is working because I am NOT dieting. I don't count calories or measure portions. I DO eat sensibly, but I don't feel like I'm really depriving myself of anything. There's no "I can't eat that until I'm done with this diet" mindset. As far as exercise, kudos to Coach JC!!! He truly is an expert at what he does. He recognizes my capacities and safely pushes me to the limits. I am stunned at what I am able to do physically in such a short period of time. Every day I feel

stronger and more flexible. I can walk and stand for extended periods without fatigue. My feet don't hurt like they did. My blood pressure has dropped markedly. My clothes are falling off. People tell me I look healthier, and I don't have to ask people to do things for me all the time. I'm sleeping better. The wounds on my shins are almost gone! My resting pulse rate is 60 beat per minute, and I can actually run!!! Okay, Usain Bolt, Olympic gold medal sprinter, may still have a stride or two on me, but I have not been able to run in YEARS!!! I can do multi-station circuit/conditioning workouts that would make many people toss their cookies! The workouts are still WORK, and always will be, but the benefits in everything else I do in my life are worth it. My deepest and heartfelt thanks to Coach JC and his staff, thank you... and finally, I'd like to thank God for showing me He's not ready for me yet..."

Tom Basler — 52 years old • www.TomBasler.com

I want to show you how working out and being fit can be fun. So many people spend endless time in the gym and are not seeing results. I want to show you how in just 27 days you can be on your way to better health and a better body. The workout is short, fun, and produces results! What you will not find in this workout is a boring drawn-out exercise regimen. Everyone's time is valuable and I realize that. This is why I developed this workout to be time efficient. If you are a stay-at-home mom, businessman, teacher, construction worker, or anything else, we will get you in, get you out, and get you fit! Everyone has a family, a job, and other obligations and commitments. Now that exercising and leading a healthy life is a priority for you, I will show you how to get your workout in while maximizing your

TIME TO GET MOVING

3

time. You don't have to spend endless hours in the gym to get results any longer. The great thing about this workout is that you can perform it wherever you are: a park, the gym, or even in the comfort of your own home. You do not need a gym membership or expensive equipment. I never prescribe anything to my clients without trying it first. I have performed this entire workout the way it is presented, and I, who have been training for twelve years, saw some great results!

The workout is for all fitness levels. I recommend that you start by using just your own body weight for each exercise. Once you feel as if you are ready for the next level, you will perform those same exercises using an external load and then increase the amount of weight that you use for each exercise. You won't see any of your traditional, drawn-out aerobic exercises like the stairclimber, elliptical, or stationary bike. I will be introducing you to our Bootcamp Tulsa style training, with the use of your own body weight for both your conditioning and strength training. I will show you how a combination of resistance training and conditioning can increase your work capacity and get your heart rate up so that you will be burning calories and fat while increasing strength. Now I will let you in on a little secret that you may not know. When you work at a higher intensity level, you actually burn more calories for a longer amount of time. Did you know that when you are done working out you continue to burn calories throughout the day? The higher the intensity of the training, the longer you will continue to burn those calories. So don't be deceived into thinking that you are cheating yourself by not spending hours in a gym on a treadmill.

Now remember, developing a new habit is never going to be easy. For us to be able to do this, I need you to turn the intensity up each and every workout. By intensity I simply mean how hard you work. These workouts will be short but intense, and the benefits will last longer. You must bring the intensity! If you are to perform for 15 seconds, then you have to go as hard as you can for 15 seconds, not 13 seconds… 15! You may look at this workout and think to yourself, "It can't be that simple!" Believe me, it will not be easy, but it definitely can be simple. The trainers at the gym don't tell you this because if they did, gyms would go out of business! People have made things so complicated that it has taken the fun out of it.

I encourage everyone to begin with the basics and then adjust the program as needed. A lot of people first look at the workout and say, "This doesn't look that bad. I can do the advanced level," and then they get started and realize that they should have begun with the basics. After the 27 days, you will have some knowledge on how to workout to maximize your time and your results. You can continue to use these workouts, design your own, or you can contact me at jc@CoachJC.com and I will personally deliver a customized workout to you every month with our online coaching program.

You are about to have the GAME PLAN to change your life!

My goal for you is that over the next 27 days you will develop good habits and make lifestyle changes that will lead to improved overall health, improved physical appearance, and improved performance so that you can live the life that you deserve and feel great in all that you do!

TIME TO GET MOVING

3

THE WARM-UP

It is very important to warm-up prior to performing any exercise routine. The warm-up is designed to prepare your body for the workout by increasing your heart rate, increasing blood flow to your muscles, and raising your core body temperature. The following warm-up routine is one of many that we use in our program. Just make sure you perform it in its entirety before beginning the daily workout. This is called a warm-up, but let me warn you by saying that most people refer to our warm-up as a workout. It is a lot more than a warm-up.

Warm-up 1

A. Stationary:

1. Jumping jacks x :30

2. Gate Swings x :15

3. Crossing jacks x :30

4. Sumo Squat x :15

B. Movement:

1. High knee with skip x :30

2. Defensive slide x :15 ea.

3. Forward walking Lunge x :30

4. Inverted Hamstring x :15

C. Ground-Based:

1. Leg Kick x :30

2. Face up crossover x :30

3. Face down crossover x :30

4. Roll to V-Sit x :15

THE SECRET TO REAL WEIGHT LOSS SUCCESS
GAME PLAN

Each day for the next 27 days you will be given your three keys to success. The Transform Your Thinking Workout, The Transform Your Body Workout, and The Transform Your Eating Workout. You must master each key for that day. Once you master the key for all three aspects, then you move on to the next day. Here is where true success lies! Once you have moved on to the next day, you still must continue to implement the components that you learned and mastered in previous workouts. So when you are on Day 27 of the game plan, you should have mastered days 1 through 26, and they should be working in your life each and everyday. Now it is time to get after it and have fun!

Make sure to visit

www.CoachJC.com

to get all of your body transformation tools!

Just 27 days to a new you!!!

Notice: The information contained in the The Secret To Real Weight Loss Success Gameplan is meant to supplement and not replace proper exercise training and nutritional guidance. All exercise poses some form of risk. I therefore advise all The Secret To Real Weight Loss Success users to take full responsibility and know your limits.

Improper form can result in injury therefore if you are unfamiliar with an exercise suggestion it is your responsibility to consult an experienced trainer to instruct you properly.

The nutritional suggestions recommended in the Game plan are not intended as a substitute for any dietary regimen prescribed by your physician. These suggestions are not intended to cure or treat any disease or illnesses.

The Secret To Real Weight Loss Success, JJC Enterprises, and the authors disclaim any liability or loss in connection with the use of this system, it's programs and advice herein.

TIME TO GET MOVING

3

Day One

THE SECRET TO REAL WEIGHT LOSS SUCCESS

You Must Want It! – Desire

How much do you really desire for change in your life? How much do you desire to lose weight and get healthy? Remember, it all starts with desire! That is the one thing that I cannot give you.

Now, I want you to ask yourself these few questions. Write down your answers and be as specific and honest with yourself as you possibly can.

1. What is it that I really desire? _____

    _____

2. How much do I really desire this? _____

    _____

3. When do I desire this by? _____

    _____

4. Who do I know also desires this? _____

    _____

5. What is the purpose? Why is it that you do what you do?

    _____

The purpose is what will drive you, what is going to keep you motivated, and what is going to make this dream, this desire, become a reality. Without a purpose you will not succeed!

THE GAME PLAN

1

Day One

TRANSFORM YOUR EATING

When Was the Last Time You Ate?

This is always such a popular topic with our clients who are trying to lose weight. When I tell them that they should be eating every two to three hours they think that I'm crazy! You may be thinking the same thing. Most Americans are use to eating only two or three meals a day. Eating every two to three hours is one of the most beneficial things you can do for both overall health and body composition. When you feed your body small frequent meals you will speed up your metabolism and help balance out your blood sugar, which will enable your body to burn off some extra calories. So, starting today you need to begin to eat every two to three hours. Okay, I know you are probably thinking, how am I going to do that? Here is how:

Start by eating five meals each day: breakfast, lunch, and dinner with a snack in between each meal. Every day you will eat three meals and two or three snacks.

Eat every three hours – period! When it is time to eat, it is time to eat. I don't care what time it is, if it has been three hours, you need to eat.

Eat smaller meals. Never eat until you are full, just eat until you are content. We will address portion sizes on day three.

Yes, it is as simple as that! Get after it… and oh yeah, have fun!

Day One

TRANSFORM YOUR BODY Today you will perform each exercise for 10 sec, rest for 20 sec, then go directly to the next exercise. Perform each exercise starting with exercise 1 and finishing with exercise 8. This equals 1 set and should take you 4 minutes. Once you complete set 1, rest for 90 sec and then perform a second set.

1 Jumping Jacks
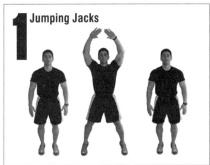

2 Push Ups
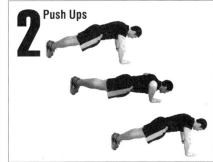

3 Jumping Jacks
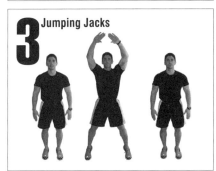

4 Counter Balance Squat
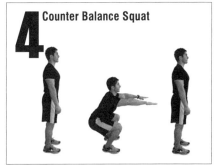

5 Jumping Jacks
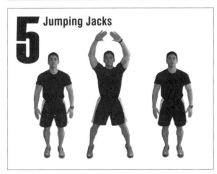

6 Push Ups
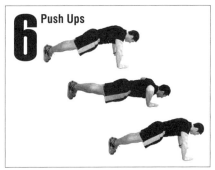

7 Jumping Jacks
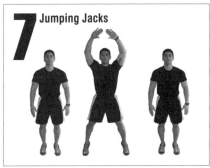

8 Counter Balance Squat
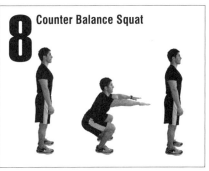

Day
Two

THE SECRET
TO REAL WEIGHT LOSS SUCCESS

What's Your Plan of Action? – Game Plan

I want you to ask yourself a question: what do you need to do on a daily basis to follow the game plan? You have the game plan in your hands; now, I want you to put together your own game plan. Your game plan is going to detail how you are going to follow this game plan. Be specific! What time of the day will you read your transformation for the day? What time of the day will you do your physical workout? What steps are you going to take to follow your nutrition plan? Write it down and follow it on a daily basis. Be as specific as possible by listing the exact times, locations, and step-by step-approach that you will take to get it done.

Today, develop your personal game plan. This should be a written itinerary of when you will do each daily component to transform your life forever.

Day
Two

TRANSFORM YOUR EATING

Measure your results

Today for your transformation, I want you to take your measurements. Okay, I know this has nothing to do with your eating, but you will see why this is so important. A lot of people beat themselves up because they do not think they are making improvements. Most of the time, they are progressing, but they don't realize it because they haven't been tracking it. I believe in measurements for a few reasons. First of all, it assures you that your plan is working, or if it is not, then you need to change something. Secondly, it can help you track your progress and allow you to look back and see where you began. Here are the measurements I want you to take.

All measurements and pictures are to be done on the first day of starting the game plan!

BEFORE	AFTER
Date:	*Date:*
Neck:	**Neck:**
Chest:	**Chest:**
Waist:	**Waist:**
Hips:	**Hips:**
Thighs : R L	**Thighs : R L**
Calves:	**Calves:**
Upper Arm:	**Upper Arm:**
Body Weight (lbs):	**Body Weight (lbs):**

*Be sure to measure the same locations, using the same measuring tool.

THE GAME PLAN

2

Day Two

BEFORE / AFTER PICTURES

Measure your results

BEFORE

Place photo here

AFTER

Place photo here

Day Two

TRANSFORM YOUR BODY Today, just like yesterday you will perform each exercise for 10 sec, rest for 20 sec, then go directly to the next exercise. Perform each exercise starting with exercise 1 and finishing with exercise 8. This equals 1 set and should take you 4 minutes. Once you complete set 1, rest for 90 sec and then perform a second set.

1. Crossing Jacks

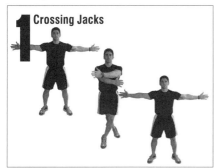

2. Negative Push Ups
(Take 5 seconds on the way down.)

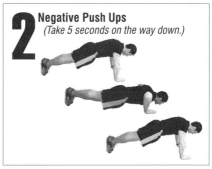

3. Crossing Jacks

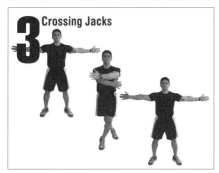

4. Split Squat
(Perform the movement on each leg for the designated time frame.)

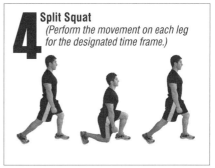

5. Jumping Jacks

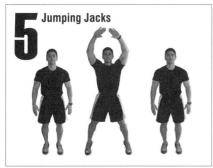

6. Inverted Row

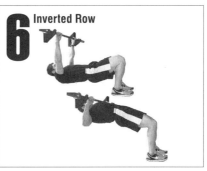

7. Jumping Jacks

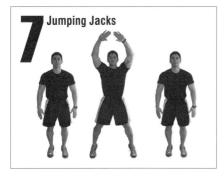

8. Split Squat
(Perform the movement on each leg for the designated time frame.)

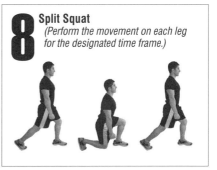

Day Three

THE SECRET TO REAL WEIGHT LOSS SUCCESS

DON'T Accept Failure

Don't Accept Failure Any More!

Failure is not an option. Today and from here on out, you will establish the no-quit mentality; the no-quit attitude.

Today for your transformation, you will draw up a contract. This contract will be between you and you. Okay, I know that seems silly, but I am serious! This contract will be a declaration that you will finish and that you will finish strong!

Today, you will sign a contract stating that you will complete this entire 27-day game plan. You will finish it! In this contract, you will also set a deadline for yourself. When will you have it completed by? Hint: it should be 24 days from now! Once you draft and sign this contract, I want you to give a copy to your accountability partner and file one for yourself.

Now get focused on it. Never quit! Start today and begin to allow your vision to expand! Here is the contract that you will use:

1. _____

2. _____

3. _____

"I hereby state that I will abide by my goals listed above. This contract is between me and me. I know that I can do it! I know that I will achieve them! There is no stopping me! I have the discipline, determination, and the will to achieve all of my goals! From this day forward I consider it done! I will complete my goals by _____(Date)"

Signature_____ Date_____

Day
Three   TRANSFORM YOUR EATING

How much are you eating?

We are not talking about counting calories here. Who has time to count calories? What we are talking about is how much are you eating at each meal? What do your portion sizes look like? You have probably heard that a portion should be the size of a deck of cards or the size of your palm. That is a great rule of thumb and the simplest way to control how many calories you are consuming. I train athletes for a living so I am really big on visualization. Just visualize it! What does a portion size look like? I like to use the ball analogy. If you are trying to lose weight, your portion size will never be the size of a basketball or even the size of a volleyball. In America, our portion sizes have become distorted. You go out to eat and you receive a meal that is enough for three people instead of just you. What do you do? You eat it; all of it. Everywhere you turn, people are encouraging you to upsize or supersize because you can save a few pennies. Not any more! From here on out, your health and your desired body are more important than a few cents. When you go out to eat at a restaurant, I want you to ask the server for a to-go box before you even receive your meal. When your meal arrives, leave only your portion size on the plate and box the rest up for later. I am actually helping you to save money because now you have a couple more meals for later! Portion control is a huge component, and you must master it if you want to take control of your health and look and feel great again.

Okay, now let's go back to the ball analogy. Start to visualize a baseball or a tennis ball; this will be the size of your meat, poultry, or fish serving. This will also be the size of your fruit servings and vegetable servings. Now, I want you to picture a half of a baseball. This will be the size of your carbohydrate serving. With salad dressing, peanut butter, and other dressings, just think of a golf ball. These different-sized balls should give

THE GAME PLAN

3

you a visual reference for serving sizes. Starting today at every meal, you must eat just one right-size portion of each food.

Ideally, every person's portion size should be based on his or her gender, activity levels, body type, body fat, and calorie needs, but for now, just keep it the size of a ball – as long as you pick the right size ball! Transform your eating today by transforming your portion sizes.

Day Three

TRANSFORM YOUR BODY Today, just like yesterday you will perform each exercise starting with 1 and finishing with 8. Today you will perform each exercise for 15 sec, and rest for 20 sec. Perform 2 sets with 90 sec in between sets. Remember, you must go as hard as you can for that 15 sec. Bring the Intensity!

1 Long Striders
(Exaggerate the movement with big strides!)

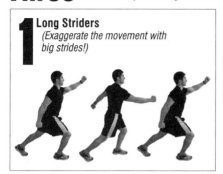

2 Push Ups

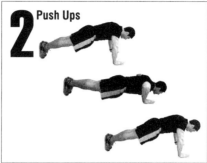

3 Crossing Jacks

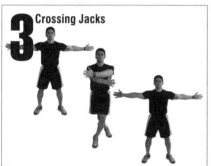

4 Forward Lunge
(Alternate legs like you are walking. Perform an even amount on each leg.)

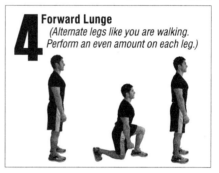

5 Long Striders
(Exaggerate the movement with big strides!)

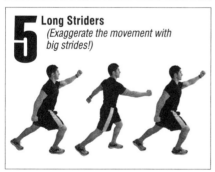

6 Pull Ups
(Beginners can perform jumping pull ups. Jump up to the top position and control the way down, then repeat.)

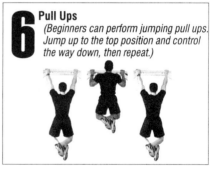

7 Crossing Jacks

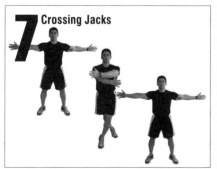

8 Forward Lunge
(Alternate legs like you are walking. Perform an even amount on each leg.)

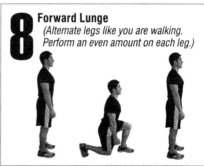

Day
Four

THE SECRET
TO REAL WEIGHT LOSS SUCCESS

DISCOVER The Power of The Mind

Today, it is time to start dreaming big once again!

What dreams have you given up on?

Today I want you to write down those dreams, and I want you to place this sheet of paper near your bed. You will say these dreams out loud every night for the next 24 days before you go to sleep and again first thing when you awake.

What does your dream body look like? What would make you feel good about yourself again?

Remember, a dream without action will always just be a dream. Start to see that image of you being successful. You must see the final product! Don't see yourself as being fat any more or unfit any more. Don't see yourself any more as being broke! By the time these 27 days are complete, you will be on your way to making those dreams a true reality. This day is dedicated to dreaming big again and developing that mental picture of what you will look like. Remember to make it as definite and specific as possible. Remember what it is that you desire!

Transform your thinking today by writing down those dreams and saying those dreams out loud every night before you go to sleep and first thing in the morning.

Day Four

TRANSFORM YOUR EATING

Get Those Veggies!

I feel like your grandma: "Don't forget to eat your vegetables!" You have probably been hearing this reminder your entire life; there is a reason for it. Vegetables are your source of life! Do you want to live long? Eat veggies! Do you want to lose weight? Eat veggies! Do you want to get stronger? Eat veggies! I don't care what your goal is you must eat vegetables. Vegetables have too many benefits to name them all here, but I have listed a few off the top of my head:

- Provide micronutrients that are low in fat and calories

- Provide minerals and vitamins to support function and energy

- Provide phytochemicals for proper physiological functioning

- Provide balanced alkaline levels to the blood

- Provide dietary fiber

- Provide nutrients that fight free radicals and cancer

Here is the cool thing! A lot of research shows a correlation of vegetable intake and fat loss. Listen, no one can argue with this key to success. To keep it simple: you have to eat your vegetables each day. Starting today, you will eat a minimum of one serving of vegetables with each meal. Therefore, you will be getting at least five servings of vegetables a day since you are eating every two to three hours. You will see what I really mean by greens when I give you my top superfoods. For now, go get those greens!

Transform your eating by increasing your intake of greens today!

THE GAME PLAN

4

Day Four

TRANSFORM YOUR BODY Today, just like yesterday you will perform each exercise starting with 1 and finishing with 8. Today you will perform each exercise for 15 sec, and rest for 20 sec. Perform 2 sets with 90 sec in between sets. Remember, you must go as hard as you can for that 15 sec. Bring the Intensity!

1 High Knees
(This is just like running in place. Get those knees up!)

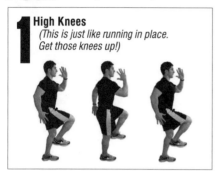

2 Dips

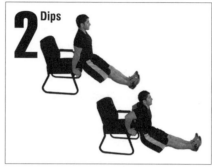

3 High Knees
(This is just like running in place. Get those knees up!)

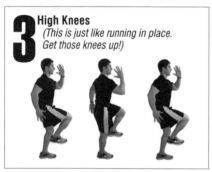

4 Swings
(This is a continual movement using a weighted object of choice.)

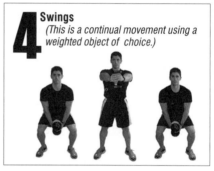

5 High Knees
(This is just like running in place. Get those knees up!)

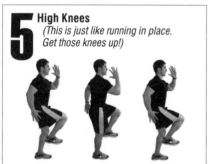

6 Dips

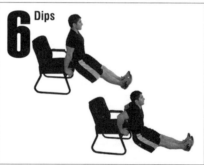

7 High Knees
(This is just like running in place. Get those knees up!)

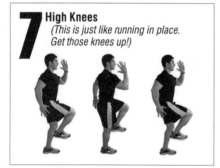

8 Swings
(This is a continual movement using a weighted object of choice.)

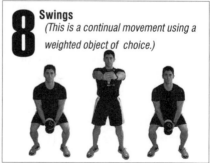

Day Five

**THE SECRET
TO REAL WEIGHT LOSS SUCCESS**

DON'T Make Excuses

You will transform your thinking today by no longer making excuses in your life.

Start today to eliminate excuses from your life and your vocabulary. Start today to eliminate blame from your life and your vocabulary.

Today, I want you to listen to yourself when you speak. Are you taking responsibility for your actions or are you putting blame on someone else? You need to begin to do this at work with your co-workers, at home with your family, and throughout your daily activities. Listen to yourself! Today, you will begin to take responsibility for your life and no longer make excuses. This is a hard thing to do, and the only way to master it is to listen to yourself when you speak. When you are about to speak negatively or make an excuse, just don't do it! If you do, then correct it right there by rephrasing what you said so that it is positive. You will transform your thinking by eliminating excuses from your life. Here are a few keys to your success.

- Have confidence in yourself and what you are doing. You have the best game plan!

- Seize the opportunity to transform your life forever. Now is your time!

- Learn from your mistakes and focus on your strengths!

- Be honest with yourself. Take responsibility for your life and make no more excuses.

THE GAME PLAN

5

Day Five

TRANSFORM YOUR EATING

Carbs Are Not From The Devil!

Are you one of those people who hears the word carbs and you automatically think, "those are bad?" Let me start by stating that all carbohydrates are not bad and your body needs them to survive and function properly. It makes a difference what kind of carbs you are eating and when are you eating them. See, most people are addicted to the wrong kinds of carbs like sweets and processed carbs. These kinds of carbs lack the nutritional value that you need but are high in calories to add to fat gain. The obvious carbs that are detrimental to your health and physique are the ones like soda, cookies, crackers, cakes, candies, etc. However, there are others that are silent assassins and are not so obvious like breads, pastas, and potatoes. These silent assassins are not horrible, but you can do better by making sure you are eating whole grain and whole wheat rather than white breads and pastas.

We always tell our clients that those silent assassin carbs are earned. If you want to eat those starchy carbs, you must exercise first and then only eat them after your workout.

GOOD CARBS *high fiber and low glycemic*	BAD CARBS *high in sugar with empty calories*
Fruits	Most Breakfast Cereals
Veggies	Soda
Whole Grain Breads	Fruit Juice
Whole Grain Pasta	Bagels
Whole Grain Cereal	Muffins
Whole Grain Rice	Crackers
Sweet Potatoes	Sugary Desserts
Whole Oats	Doughnuts
Grain Cereals	Ice Cream

If you want to lose fat, then you must control your carbohy-drate intake. We are not talking about a low-carb diet here. I am simply talking about being able to distinguish between a good carb and a bad carb and knowing when you should be eating them. Now, don't forget that veggies and fruits are also carbs and that veggies are free game. Eat away! Starting today, you will only eat bad carbs on your "free" day, which we will talk about on Day 10. Also, you will only eat starchy carbs as a reward after exercising. If you don't exercise, you will get your carbs from eating fruits and veggies.

Transform your eating today by mastering your carb intake!

THE GAME PLAN

5

Day Five

TRANSFORM YOUR BODY Today you will perform each exercise starting with 1 and finishing with 8 but we are going to kick the intensity up a little. Today you will perform each exercise for 15 sec. and rest for only 15 sec. Perform 2 sets with 90 sec in between sets. Burn those calories! Bring the Intensity!

1 Jumping Jacks

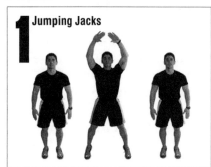

2 Squat to Press

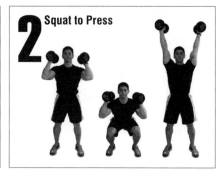

3 High Knees
(This is just like running in place. Get those knees up!)

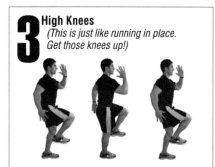

4 Pull Ups
(Beginners can perform jumping pull ups. Jump up to the top position and control the way down, then repeat.)

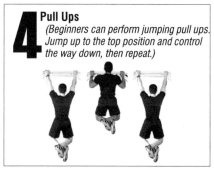

5 Crossing Jacks

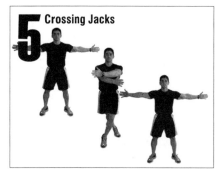

6 Reverse Lunge
(Make sure to alternate legs each rep!)

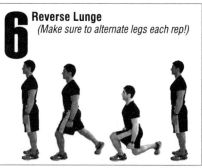

7 Long Striders
(Exaggerate the movement with big strides!)

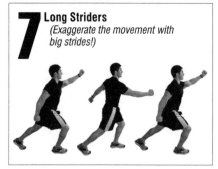

8 Close Grip Push Ups

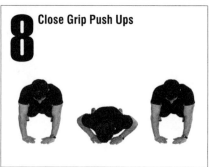

Day Six

THE SECRET
TO REAL WEIGHT LOSS SUCCESS

DECIDE To Let Negativity Go

Your challenge today is to eliminate negativity from your life!

Today, you will make a list of negative thoughts that you have about yourself. You will then list five areas of negativity in your life that you feel are holding you back or hindering you from achieving ultimate success. It could be something that robs your time; it could be a family member, a friend, or a co-worker who continues to tell you that you can't lose weight; maybe it is the media that continues to bombard you with negative thoughts and perceptions.

For the next 22 days, I want you to completely disassociate yourself with these things because they will drain your energy and distract you from your ultimate goal.

Now, you will list five positive things about yourself, and starting today, you will ask your accountability partner and one other person whom you trust to tell you at least one of those things every time that you speak with them. Also, begin to tell yourself these five positive things about yourself throughout every day from here on out.

THE GAME PLAN

6

Day Six

TRANSFORM YOUR EATING

Have You been Drinking?

With any client who is looking to lose weight, we always ask them the same question, "Have you been drinking?" This is because most people don't realize how many empty calories they are consuming throughout the day from the beverages they drink. Consequently, we always take a look at what he or she is drinking. Calories can add up quickly if you are dinking soda, fruit juices, coffee with creamer, energy drinks, beer, or all those other sugary drinks. Your transformation for today is the zero calorie rule! Starting today you will not drink any beverages with more than zero calories. So yes, that is pretty much just water and real tea. I realize that this may be advice that you have heard before, but remember, this is a game plan and this is part two that you need to master in your nutrition. Zero-Calorie Beverages! The amount of sugar that food manufacturers use in beverages is crazy. One can of soda has about ten teaspoons of sugar... that's ridiculous! So, starting today your goal is two-fold: to eliminate these beverages from your daily consumption and to drink more water. Did you know that your body is made up of 60 percent water? Water is essential for your body to perform at its optimal level, and most people don't realize how important water is for fat loss. We always advise our clients to get at least eight glasses (or half of their body weight in ounces) of water a day. On days that you exercise, you should get at least 16 glasses of water per day.

*If you are exercising outside in extreme heat you may need to consume a sports drink that contains electrolytes, carbohydrates, and minerals, as water will not replenish those important minerals that you are sweating out at that time.

Day Six

TRANSFORM YOUR BODY Today you will perform each exercise starting with 1 and finishing with 8. Just like yesterday, you will perform each exercise for 15 sec. and rest for 15 sec. Perform 2 sets with 90 sec in between sets. How bad do you want it?

1 Mountain Climbers
(Continue to alternate legs for the entire time.)

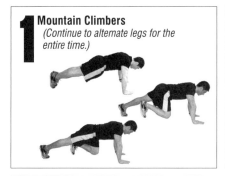

2 Inverted Row

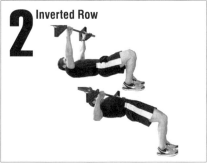

3 High Knees
(This is just like running in place. Get those knees up!)

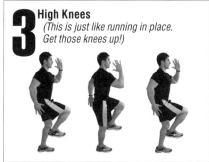

4 Step Up
(Alternate legs throughout the entire time - up, down, down, up.)

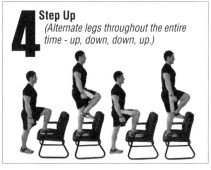

5 Inverted Row

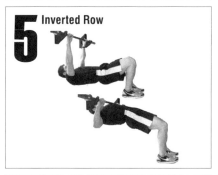

6 High Knees
(This is just like running in place. Get those knees up!)

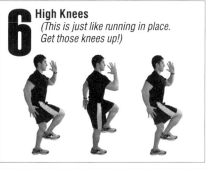

7 Step Up
(Alternate legs throughout the entire time - up, down, down, up.)

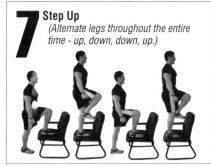

8 Mountain Climbers
(Continue to alternate legs for the entire time.)

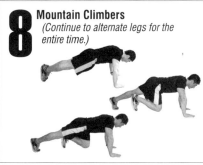

Day
Seven
THE SECRET
TO REAL WEIGHT LOSS SUCCESS

DETERMINE Your Attitude

Today you will develop your attitude!

Remember, this is not cockiness, it is confidence. Starting today, I want you to know and take ownership of the fact that you will accomplish your ultimate goal. No doubt!

Determine that you will not feel sorry for yourself any longer. You will stop worrying about not accomplishing your goal. Begin to know that the results you desire will come.

Remember, your attitude reflects who you are! Your attitude from today going forward is, "I will not quit until I get there."

Begin today, to no longer look at where you are, but rather, at where you are going.

Now is your time!

Day
Seven TRANSFORM YOUR EATING

Where Is Your Complete Protein?

When most people think about protein, they think about building muscle. Protein is essential for building muscle, but protein also performs more important jobs for the body then just building muscle. Protein is not just for bodybuilders!

Protein is an important nutrient needed by everyone on a daily basis. Protein is made up of essential and non-essential amino acids. These amino acids are the "building blocks" for healthy bodies. Besides building muscle, protein has a number of different roles in the body, including the following:

- Helps repair body cells

- Assists in building and repairing muscles and bones

- Provides a source of energy

- Manages many of the important processes in the body related to metabolism

The body can produce non-essential amino acids from other amino acids in the body. However, the body is not able to make essential amino acids, and the only way to get them is to eat high-quality protein. Protein sources that contain all of the essential amino acids are called complete proteins. These complete proteins are the ones that you will eat with each meal. Women should be getting 15 to 25 grams of protein per meal and men should be getting 30 to 50 grams of protein per meal.

THE GAME PLAN

7

Complete Protein Sources:

- Lean meats (chicken, turkey, venison, beef, bison)

- Fish (salmon, tilapia, halibut, tuna)

- Eggs (Omega 3)

- Low fat dairy (cottage cheese, low fat cheese, yogurt)

- Protein Supplements (whey, casein, milk blends)

Starting today, you must have a serving of a complete protein at each meal!

Day Seven

TRANSFORM YOUR BODY

R E C O V E R Y

Today you will be off from performing exercises so that your body can rest. Today you will stay active by doing something that you enjoy. I want for you to stay active doing something that you enjoy for at least 30 min!

TRY

- taking a walk
- playing at the park with your kids
- taking a bike ride
- playing a game

Have fun and get ready to kick it up tomorrow in your workout!

N O T E S :

THE GAME PLAN

7

Day
Eight
THE SECRET
TO REAL WEIGHT LOSS SUCCESS

DO Change Your Thinking

What is your four-minute mile barrier?

What things in your thinking have been holding you back from ultimate success?

Choose today to let go of this kind of thinking!

In what areas of your life have you not been prosperous?

Make a decision today that you will be prosperous in these areas from here on out. Today, I want you to write down all of these areas on three pieces of paper and make them visible in three different places that you visit on a daily basis. For example, you could place them in your car, near your refrigerator, and in the bathroom. Every time you see these sheets, I want you to state, out loud, those areas that you will prosper in.

Remove the negative thinking and negative influences in your life. Decide to break through your mental barriers today just like Roger Bannister did with the mile run! Today, your transformation is to make a decision to change your thinking for good!

Day Eight

TRANSFORM YOUR EATING

You Need Fat?

Okay, I know what you are saying, "Fat is not good! I am trying to lose fat! Why do I want to eat more fat?" I could write a whole chapter on the importance of fat for your body. There are three classifications of fat: saturated fat, monounsaturated fat, and polyunsaturated fat. About 30 percent of your daily nutrients should come from fat. Additionally, you should get a fairly equal percentage (33% of your fat intake) from each of the three different kinds of fat. Most people get enough saturated fat daily, so I want you to start getting more monounsaturated and polyunsaturated fats throughout the day.

I have listed some great sources of these fats below:

Monounsaturated: Olive Oil, Nuts and Nut Butters, Avocados

Polyunsaturated: Fish oil, Flax seeds, Vegetable Oils

Here are just a few of the benefits of incorporating good fats into your daily routine:

- Lower cholesterol
- Anti-cancer effects
- Antioxidants
- Anti-inflammatory effects
- Quicker recovery time
- Improved stamina and endurance
- Increased energy
- Faster Metabolism

Lose fat by eating fat! It's time to go fishing!

THE GAME PLAN

8

Day Eight

TRANSFORM YOUR BODY Today you will perform each exercise starting with 1 and finishing with 8 but we are going to kick the intensity up a little from week one. Today you will perform each exercise for 20 sec, and rest for only 15 sec. Perform 2 sets through all 8 exercises with 90 sec of rest in between sets. Get after it!

1 Burpees

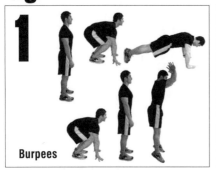

2 Squat to Press

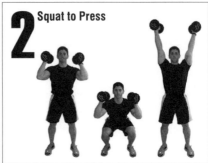

3 Split Squat Jumps
(Make sure to alternate legs each rep!)

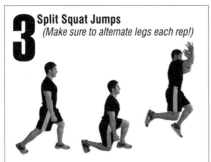

4 Defensive Slide
(Perform 5 yards each side back and forth for the designated time.)

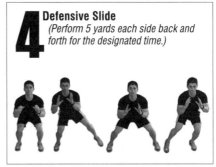

5 Squat to Press

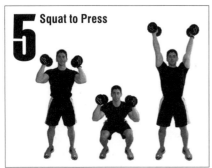

6 Split Squat Jumps
(Make sure to alternate legs each rep!)

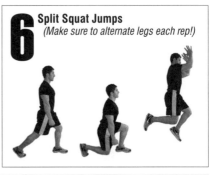

7 Defensive Slide
(Perform 5 yards each side back and forth for the designated time.)

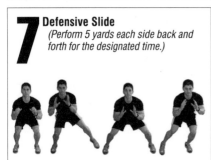

8 Burpees

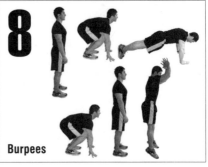

Day
Nine

THE SECRET
TO REAL WEIGHT LOSS SUCCESS

DON'T Fear Failing

Today you will eliminate the fear from your life!

What has fear kept you from achieving in your life? What is it that you are afraid of? What have you failed to start because you were afraid you might fail?

Have you been paralyzed right where you were because you were afraid of failing? From today on, the fear of failure is no longer your worst enemy. Starting today, you are going to go and attack that thing that you have feared. From here on out, you will begin to take risks in life. The biggest fear people face is the fear of failure. This fear will rob you of your dreams. You will now address the fear that has crippled your goals and has kept you from accomplishing your dreams. You will begin to dream once again, and you will no longer allow fear to keep you from dreaming. I want you to say out loud to yourself "I will no longer live a mediocre life!"

Your goal is to detect this fear in your life, learn how to address it, and overcome it. You will do this by simply dismissing it and moving forward. This step alone will enable you to be one step closer to accomplishing the body of which you always dreamed. If this fear arises, ask yourself a question: "What is the worst that could happen if this fear of failure became a reality in my life?" When you think about it, the worst that could happen isn't really that bad. Then ask yourself, "What is the best outcome that could happen in my life once I disable the fear of failure?" That best outcome will always outweigh the worst thing. Now go and chase your dreams. Go and get that body that you want, need, and ultimately deserve.

THE GAME PLAN

9

Day
Nine TRANSFORM YOUR EATING

Plan and Prepare

You probably have heard the saying, "If you fail to plan, then you are planning to fail." This is so true when it comes to your nutrition. You have to start planning and preparing! You must know what you are going to eat at each meal and at what time you are going to eat that meal. You must also know what you are going to eat the next day and plan for that as well. With your job, all your commitments, and all your responsibilities, this is vital for your success. This will take a commitment on your part. You will need to write down what you will be eating at each meal the following day; then you will need to make sure you have access to those foods.

Here are a few tips to help you in your planning and preparing.

- When you cook, cook a little extra for another meal. For example, if you are grilling chicken, grill some extra for future meals in the next few days.

- Use Tupperware containers to bring food on the road with you.

- Chop your veggies once a week and keep them in baggies or containers to save time later.

- Utilize shaker bottles and blenders. These are always convenient when you are on the road.

- Keep mixed nuts, fruit and other healthy snacks with you at all times.

For your transformation today, you will start to plan and prepare each meal and come up with creative ways to maximize your time. Once you master this, watch how easy this whole nutritional lifestyle change becomes!

Day Nine

TRANSFORM YOUR BODY Today you will perform each exercise starting with 1 and finishing with 8. You will perform each exercise for 20 sec and rest for 15 sec. Perform 2 sets through with 90 sec rest in between sets.

1. Push up to Row

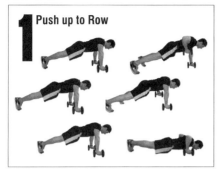

2. Side Lunge
(Perform each side for the designated time.)

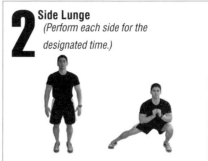

3. Body Builders

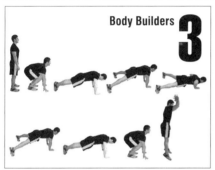

4. Squat to Press

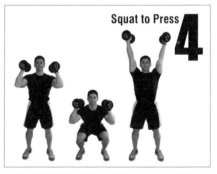

5. Squat Jumps

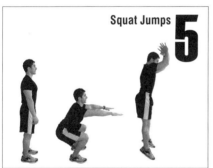

6. Body Builders

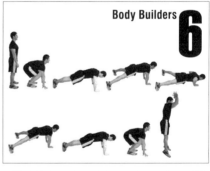

7. Inverted Row

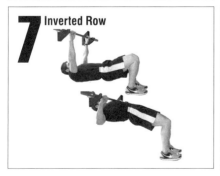

8. Side Lunge
(Perform each side for the designated time.)

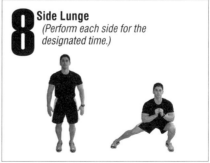

Day Ten

THE SECRET TO REAL WEIGHT LOSS SUCCESS

DECIDE to Let Go of the Past

What are those things from your past that have been holding you back from experiencing ultimate happiness in your life? For your transformation today, you will open the bag of past memories and events and sort through it! Throw away any of the things that you do not need any more. Only keep those things that you need to go on with your future.

Remember, that the past is the past! You can only control the effect that the past has on you right now. Today, you will stop trying to make the past something that it was not. If you did not accomplish the things that you wanted to in the past, stop beating yourself up, release it, and start your future free of guilt, fear, and anxiety! If you stay stuck in the past, then you will continue to repeat those past patterns and never see the results you desire. Transform yourself today by setting yourself free of these past patterns and by looking to the future ahead of you. You will start today by taking responsibility for the choices that you make today. Now is your time to be your best! Let go of what is holding you back; being free is a great feeling. Choose today to let your past go. Begin to write the script for your present and future!

The sky is the limit! Time for you to fly!

Day
Ten

TRANSFORM YOUR EATING

Plan to Cheat!

It is okay to enjoy the foods that you like. To succeed and see optimal results, you must eat the foods that you like! You just cannot eat them every day. I will give you two options: you can have a free day once a week or you can eat free 10 percent of the time. This book is not about being perfect but about making a few lifestyle changes. Life is all about enjoyment, and you will see that once you conquer your eating, you will enjoy life even more. To have "free-will meals" or a "cheat day" is important from a psychological perspective. If you choose option one, then you will pick one day a week that you are free to have the foods that are not on your plan. Please understand that this means that you can have some foods that are not on your plan, but you still must stay within your portion sizes. This option works for a lot of our clients and it works best for me.

With option two, you will plan to break the plan 10 percent of the time throughout the week. So, let's say you are eating five times a day for seven days a week, which means 35 meals for the entire week. With a little math skill, we can figure out that 10 percent of 35 is 3.5, so that means you can have three meals each week that don't follow the plan. This option works for a lot of our clients, but you must be very careful that your 10 percent doesn't turn into 20 or 30 percent. Today, your transformation is to plan your weekly free day or free meals and schedule what you are going to eat for those meals or day. The rest of the time, stay true to the game plan!

THE GAME PLAN

10

Day Ten

TRANSFORM YOUR BODY Today you will perform each exercise starting with 1 and finishing with 8. You will perform each exercise for 20 sec, and rest for only 15 sec. Perform 2 sets through all 8 exercises with 90 sec of rest in between sets. Remember, your goal is to get as many reps as possible for the time.

1 In and Outs
(Jump your feet out and in.)

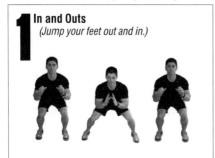

2 Rotational Push Ups
(Make sure to perform an even amount on each side. Alternate each rep.)

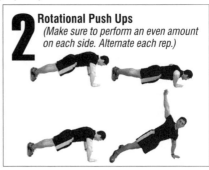

3 Squats

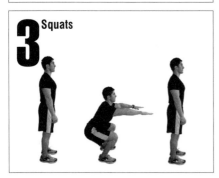

4 Burpee with Push Up

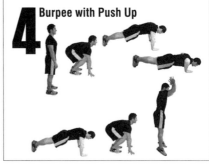

5 Pull Ups
(Beginners can perform jumping pull ups. Jump up to the top position and control the way down, then repeat.)

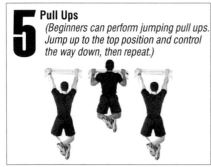

6 Step Up
(Alternate legs throughout the entire time - up, down, down, up.)

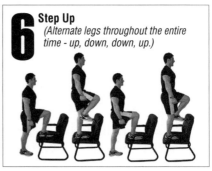

7 High Knees
(This is just like running in place. Get those knees up!)

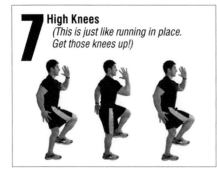

8 Swings
(This is a continual movement using a weighted object of choice.)

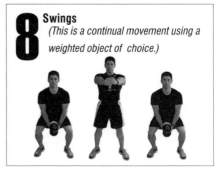

Day
Eleven
THE SECRET
TO REAL WEIGHT LOSS SUCCESS

DON'T Ever Quit

Starting today you will decide to never QUIT!

Today is when you will establish your no-quit mentality. I want you to start by telling yourself that you will not stop. This goes back to, "Why is it that I do what I do? What is your purpose?" If you really want something to work, then you have to stick with it. Don't go searching for the newest diet pill or the next fad diet. Stick with this game plan, it is proven to work and will work if you don't quit on it. Remember, the plan will not fail you! You just must make sure that you do not fail the plan.

When you feel like giving up, just remind yourself of the reasons why you are doing this. It is very important to know why you are doing what you are doing.

Starting today you will make the decision to not give up – to never quit.

Why do you do what you do? Never forget your reasons!

THE GAME PLAN

11

Day Eleven

TRANSFORM YOUR EATING

Let's Go Shopping!

If you ever want to take control of your health, you have to conquer your eating habits. If you ever want to conquer your eating habits, you have to learn how to grocery shop. I always tell my clients that it all starts at the grocery store. If you have the right foods in your house, then you should not have a problem eating right. So, today your game plan is to become the master grocery shopper. Here is how you will do that.

First, you should fill most of your cart with foods from the outside perimeter aisles. All of your fruits, veggies, and lean proteins are located in the produce and meat sections along the outside aisles. Second, you want to go to the aisles with oats, whole grains, seeds, and nuts, and pick up items such as walnuts, almonds, pecans, cashews, sunflower seeds, and flaxseeds. Just mix it up!

Next, you will get your beans! Legumes such as peas, kidney beans, chickpeas, and lentils are primarily what you want to get.

When choosing foods at the grocery store, always buy raw, fresh foods first, then frozen food, and then canned foods. Stay away from the bakery, the chip aisle, and the cookie/cracker aisle.

Always make a list and stick to it.

Here is an example of how I categorize my grocery list.

Produce – Vegetables and Fruits

- Lettuce

- Spinach

- Tomatoes

- Bell Peppers

- Cucumbers

- Bananas

Meat and Dairy

- Extra Lean Beef

- Chicken Breast

- Fish

- Eggs

- Fat-Free Cottage Cheese

- Low-Fat Yogurt

Inner Aisles

- Beans (Variety)

- Tuna

- Olive Oil

- Oats

- Flax Seeds

- Case of Spring Water

*Today I want for you to make your next grocery list, make it a fun event and remember you must master this key to be successful!

THE GAME PLAN

11

Day Eleven

TRANSFORM YOUR BODY Today you will perform each exercise starting with 1 and finishing with 8 just like you did yesterday. You will perform each exercise for 20 sec, and rest for only 10 sec. now. Perform 2 sets through all 8 exercises with 90 sec of rest in between sets.

1 High Knees
(This is just like running in place. Get those knees up!)

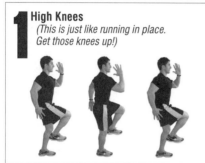

2 Squat Jumps

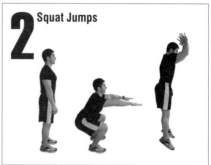

3 Defensive Slide
(Perform 5 yards each side back and forth for the designated time.)

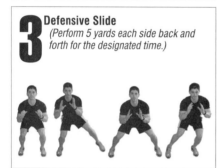

4 Curl Squat to Press

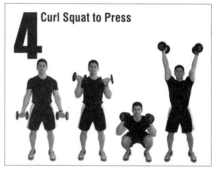

5 Forward Lunge
(Alternate legs like you are walking. Perform an even amount on each leg.)

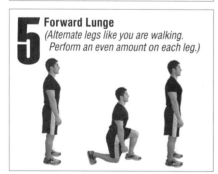

6 Long Strider
(Exaggerate the movement with big strides!)

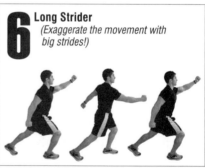

7 Rotational Push Ups
(Make sure to perform an even amount on each side. Alternate each rep.)

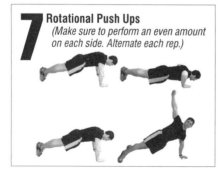

8 Squats

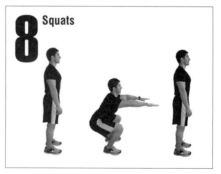

Day
Twelve
THE SECRET
TO REAL WEIGHT LOSS SUCCESS

DO Change your thinking

What is your four-minute mile barrier?

Today's goal is for you to Change Your Thinking once and for all! Starting today, you will refuse to let others determine your outcome. You will no longer allow others to put limits on your life. Starting today, you will determine your own future and your own destiny. Make the decision that you are in control and that the media, your family members, friends, magazines, other books, co-workers, etc. are not in control. It is time to take the lid off your life and to start to break some records like Roger Bannister. It is time to believe that you can do it. It is time to remove all fear and doubt from your life. Now is your time! Now is your time to think big!

What is your four-minute mile barrier? Today, for your transformation you will…

- Write your barriers down.

- Change the "I can't" to "I will"

- Remove the negative thinking!

- Decide to break through your mental barriers!

THE GAME PLAN

12

Day Twelve TRANSFORM YOUR EATING

Time to Clean Shop

That's right, it is time to clean shop! Today you will clean out your pantry and your refrigerator. This step is when most people make a mistake; they keep the bad foods in the house! Why tempt yourself? A lot of people do not have the self-control to refrain from eating certain things, and by keeping it in the house, it just makes the process more difficult. Today you will take a few steps to help you with this. The first step is to get a large black trash bag. The second step is to go through the pantry and refrigerator, and then throw the following items into the trash bag: cookies, candy, cakes, doughnuts, crackers, potato chips, and all other hydrogenated foods and junky sweets. Now, the third and final step is to take that trash bag and put it outside in the trash where it belongs. You will replace these foods with the great ones that you bought when we took our trip to the grocery store. This is always such a tough step for people to take. So I ask you, How bad do you really want it?

Day Twelve

TRANSFORM YOUR BODY Today you will perform each exercise starting with 1 and finishing with 8. You will perform each exercise for 20 sec, and rest for 10 sec. Perform 2 sets through all 8 exercises with 90 sec of rest in between sets.

Body Builders 1

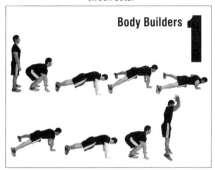

Lunge with Chop 2
(Make sure to perform each side for the designated time.)

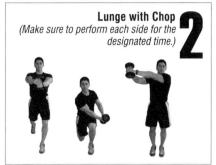

3 Negative Push Ups
(Take 5 seconds on the way down.)

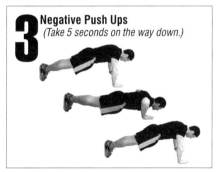

4 High Knees
(This is just like running in place. Get those knees up!)

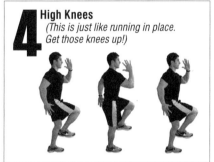

5 Inverted Row

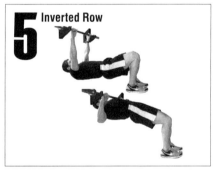

6 Squat Jumps

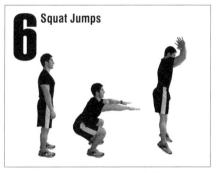

7 In and Outs
(Jump your feet out and in.)

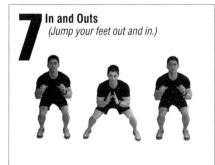

8

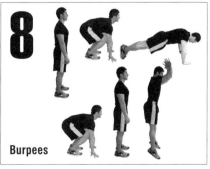

Burpees

Day
Thirteen

THE SECRET
TO REAL WEIGHT LOSS SUCCESS

DO Think Big

Today's key for your success is to think big!

Expect big things! Starting today, do everything you do in excellence. To master today, you have to change your mindset. Start by taking the limits off your life! Start to say things like, "I can lose more weight! I can get a better job! My marriage can be the best! I can make more money! I can have the body that I have always wanted!" You have to believe in yourself!

Today you will start faking! Fake it until you make it. So, you want to be healthy? Start acting like you are healthy. Do you want to be fit? How would you act if you were fit? Start acting like that! If you want to change where you are in life, then start faking it until you make it. Start acting how you would act if you were already at your ultimate goal.

Transform your thinking today by starting to fake it until you make it and begin to think as big as you possibly can!

Day
Thirteen TRANSFORM YOUR EATING

Time To Keep a Journal

Starting today you will begin to keep a journal or food log of your daily eating habits. You will write down everything that you put into your mouth and the time that you do. This will be your way to hold yourself accountable.

Here are three keys to help you successfully keep a food log:

1. Would you prefer to carry a notebook and a pen so that you can pull it out anywhere, or would you rather log your food log online? Several free online food logs are available. You must find what works for you and just do it!

2. You must write down everything. Anything that you drink or eat must be logged. Try to be as specific as possible with the size and what kind. Everything gets logged!

3. Examine your results. Did you stay true to the game plan? How about your portion sizes? Did you get your complete protein that meal? If consistent trends start to show up in your food log, it will be easier for you to make adjustments to reach your goals.

Start Journaling Today!

THE GAME PLAN

13

Day Thirteen

TRANSFORM YOUR BODY Today you will perform each exercise starting with 1 and finishing with 8. Perform each exercise for 20 sec, and rest for 10 sec. Perform 2 sets through all 8 exercises with 90 sec. of rest in between sets. Remember, execute each exercise with perfect form and get as many reps as you can in 20 sec.!

1 Push Ups - Feet Elevated

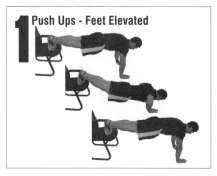

2 Split Squat Jumps
(Make sure to alternate legs each rep!)

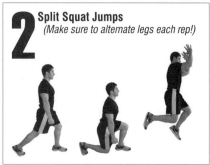

3 Mountain Climbers
(Continue to alternate legs for the entire time.)

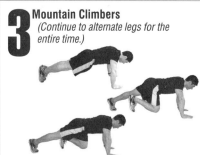

4 Pull Ups
(Beginners can perform jumping pull ups. Jump up to the top position and control the way down, then repeat.)

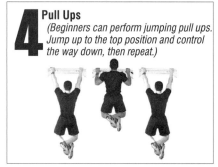

5 Side Lunge
(Perform each side for the designated time.)

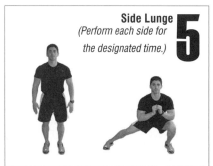

6 Body Builders

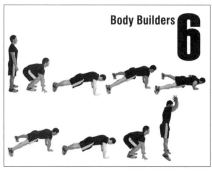

7 High Pull / Squat to Press

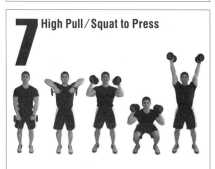

8 Side Plank
(Perform each side for the designated time.)

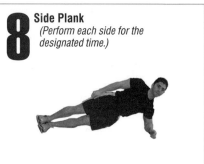

Day
Fourteen THE SECRET
TO REAL WEIGHT LOSS SUCCESS

DISCOVER Accountability

**Today you will transform your life by becoming account-
able!**

By now, you already know how important it is to be accountable. Today, you will find someone you are close to and respect
and someone you can trust. Today, you will contact them and
inform them of what you are working on if they don't already
know. Ask them if they can commit to helping you through
these last 14 days of your transformation and beyond. You will
have to be transparent with these people, so pick two people
who can really help you and who really want to see you succeed.
You will ask them to call you once a week to check up on you,
but you will also be calling them whenever you need someone
to keep you on track or to get you back on the right track.

Transform your life today by becoming accountable. Starting
today, you will contact your accountability partner at least twice
this week to allow them to make you better and help you stick to
your goals.

14

THE GAME PLAN

Day Fourteen

TRANSFORM YOUR EATING

Workout and Then Eat

You have probably heard many different ideas and suggestions about eating after you exercise. Should you? Shouldn't you? What exactly should you eat? And many more…

Eating after you exercise is crucial for you to be successful and reach your desired goals.

The bottom line is this: after long, strenuous exercise you need to refuel your body. The best way to assure that your body is properly recovering is to get a combination of protein and carbohydrates within two hours after exercise. This combination will help you to rebuild muscle tissue that is damaged during intense exercise and will help you replenish your glycogen stores. Without boring you, I want you to know the importance of this time. Look at the supplements on the market and all the money companies are making because people are figuring out the importance of a post-workout replenishing meal. The other key to post-workout recovery is to make sure that you replenish your hydration levels. I am not going to get into exactly how much food and water you need. Right now, it is just important that you are getting a meal that consists of complex carbohydrates and a lean complete protein.

Your transformation, starting today is to make sure that you are getting a meal within two hours after exercise. No excuses!

Day
Fourteen
TRANSFORM YOUR
BODY

R E C O V E R Y

Today you will be off from performing exercises so that your body can rest. Today you will stay active by doing something that you enjoy. I want for you to stay active doing something that you enjoy for at least 30 min!

TRY

- taking a walk
- playing at the park with your kids
- taking a bike ride
- playing a game

Have fun and get ready to kick it up tomorrow in your workout!

N O T E S :

14

T H E G A M E P L A N

Day
Fifteen

THE SECRET
TO REAL WEIGHT LOSS SUCCESS

DETERMINE a Sense of Urgency

If you have not already, today is your time to develop a sense of urgency. For some of you it is a matter of life or death! So what is it going to be? It is time to get out of your comfort zone and to get back in the race. Starting today, you need to feel that accomplishing your goals is a matter of life and death. True greatness is achieved from having a sense of urgency. You cannot afford to prolong your dreams and goals any longer. You owe it to yourself and your loved ones to live a long, healthy life. Are you willing to pay the price? Are you willing to do whatever it takes? We all want to have a great body and live free of diseases, but the question is, are you willing to put the time in to do whatever it takes to accomplish your dreams and goals? What is a sense of urgency? It is when you feel like you have got to do it now. It is now or never! You know that if you don't take control of it now, it is only going to get worse. This is when a sense of urgency comes into play. You must have the attitude that "I would rather be dead then to live a mediocre life." How badly do you really want it?

Transform your life and your body today by developing a true sense of urgency! Start to become truly passionate about that which you are chasing! Begin to visualize the end and what it will feel like! Make sure you hit your deadlines by taking care of business each day for the remaining 13 days and beyond! Eliminate every excuse and be proud of yourself!

Day
Fifteen TRANSFORM YOUR EATING

It's Breakfast Time!

Some people really believe that skipping breakfast may help them lose weight. Well, that is not true! Breakfast has been called the most important meal of the day for a reason. You may have heard this before, but do you know why? Your brain and central nervous system run on glucose, which is the fuel that you need to think, talk, walk, and function in most any and all activities. Let's say that the last time you eat something is at 10 p.m., then you don't eat breakfast the following morning, and wait until noon to eat. You have gone fourteen hours with nothing in your system. Your brain will be deprived and your body is going to have to work extra hard to break down any stored nutrients into a useful form, just so that your brain can function. Eating breakfast is crucial in helping you to think faster and clearer and to function properly throughout the day. So, what about losing weight and getting lean and thin? Breakfast jump-starts your metabolism. When you don't eat breakfast, your body will go into a fasting state and will not produce the proper enzymes needed to metabolize fat so that you can lose weight. The other problem with skipping breakfast or meals is that it often leads to overeating later in the day. When you allow yourself to become over-hungry, it will be harder to control what you eat later in the day. This is because it will lead to a distorted satiety feeling, meaning it's hard to determine when you're full. When this happens, people have a tendency to eat more calories then if they had eaten breakfast.

15

THE GAME PLAN

Day Fifteen

TRANSFORM YOUR BODY Today you will perform each exercise starting with 1 and finishing with 8 but we will kick the intensity up. You will now perform each exercise for 30 sec, and rest for 15 sec. Perform 2 sets through all 8 exercises with 90 sec of rest in between sets.

1 Mountain Climbers
(Continue to alternate legs for the entire time.)

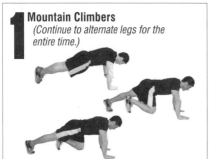

2 Swings
(This is a continual movement using a weighted object of choice.)

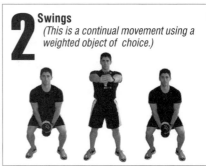

3 Plank
(Perform plank position for the designated time.)

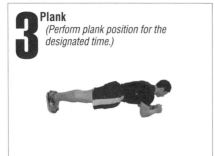

4 Curl Squat to Press

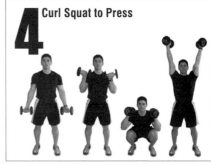

5 Defensive Slide
(Perform 5 yards each side back and forth for the designated time.)

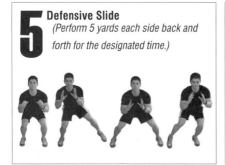

6 Side Plank
(Perform each side for the designated time.)

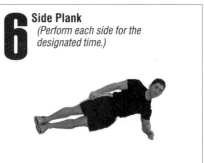

7 High Knees
(This is just like running in place. Get those knees up!)

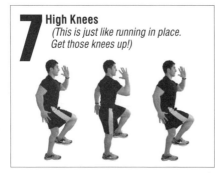

8 High Pull / Squat to Press

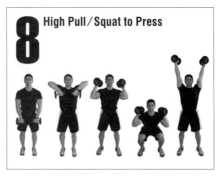

Day Sixteen

THE SECRET TO REAL WEIGHT LOSS SUCCESS

DO Get Back In The Race

Today You will Get Back in the Race!

Ask any runner and they will tell you that it is not about how you start but how you finish. If things don't start right, you can't just give up; you have to keep running. Maybe you have tried to get fit before, maybe you have tried diet after diet, maybe you have even hired a personal trainer, but you didn't see the results, so you dropped out of the race. Today, I want you to get back into the race. To finish the race you first have to start the race. I don't care what happened in the past, your new race begins today. Today is the day you get back into the race. Remember, your race is your life. Life is short and once it is over, it is over. Today, I want you to re-submit your name, put your sneakers on, and get back into the race. Once you get back in, you have a chance to win the race.

There will always be someone trying to take you back out of the race, and in the past, you may have allowed this to occur. Not any longer! When someone or circumstances threaten to take you out and steal the joy of accomplishing your goal, you can't allow it to happen. You must refuse to be knocked down; you must refuse to be knocked out. You must keep running and not look back. If you need a drink, don't even stop; instead, grab one as you keep going. Nothing slows you down and nothing takes you back out of the race.

Today for your transformation, you will vow to yourself and to your accountability partners that you will run this race with all that you have. You will commit to finishing strong! I want you to think of those things that have taken you out of the race in the past, and I want you to eliminate them from your life today. Get back in the race!

16

THE GAME PLAN

Day Sixteen TRANSFORM YOUR EATING

Coach JC's Super Foods

Many different foods are beneficial to your body in many different ways. With this plan, you will eat a wide variety of those foods. Today, I want to give you just a few that I strongly believe in. These seven super foods are foods that many people are lacking in their plan. I have seen clients make just a few lifestyle changes and see great results. This is one of those small lifestyle changes!

If you are not getting these foods on a daily basis, it is imperative that you start to incorporate them into your plan as soon as possible!

Coach JC's 7 Super Foods:

1. Mixed Berries – First of all, berries taste great! They are extremely high in nutrients, especially vitamin C and fiber. Berries are powerful antioxidants and are packed with vitamins and minerals. Research even shows that berries may help slow down the aging process, boost immunity, and protect against chronic diseases and cancers. The cool thing is that these great-tasting treats have no fat and are super low in calories!

2. Olive Oil – I love olive oil and not just because I am Italian. I was brought up pretty much drinking olive oil from the bottle. Olive oil is a monounsaturated fat packed with some great health benefits. It has some great antioxidative substances, and numerous studies show that olive oil can protect against heart disease. Olive oil helps control your LDL (bad)

cholesterol levels and helps raise your HDL (good) cholesterol levels.

3. Salmon – Salmon, a low-mercury fish, is a great source of easily digestible amino acids (proteins) that are essential components for your cells, tissues, enzymes, hormones, and almost every other body part. It is crucial for your cardio-vascular health since it is packed with omega-3 fatty acids. Salmon can help reduce blood pressure, lower cholesterol levels, and reduce the chances of a heart attack. These omega-3 fatty acids also help increase the influence of insulin, which aids in the absorption of sugar. They also help lower blood sugar levels, which has a tremendously positive influence on your metabolism. This is great news for someone who is trying to lose weight!

4. Greens – When I talk about "greens," I am talking about green foods. This group of foods includes grasses, like barley grass and wheat grass, and blue-green algae. These foods are closely associated with dark green, leafy vegetables and are high in levels of nutrients. These green foods contain a ton of the beneficial phytonutrients and have been linked to beneficial effects on cholesterol, blood pressure, immune response, and cancer prevention. This is due to their high concentrations of chlorophyll. Chlorophyll is the phytochemical that gives leaves, plants, and algae their green color. These greens are also packed with vitamins.

5. Nuts and Seeds – Nuts and seeds are some of the best plant sources of protein. They are rich in fiber and antioxidants and

16

THE GAME PLAN

also high in fat, mostly monounsaturated and polyunsatu-rated fats (the good fats). Nuts are high in calories and fat and are very calorically dense, which is why most people avoid them. They are a great snack, and most people find it very tough not to overeat them. If you can restrain yourself from overeating them, nuts and seeds need to be a part of your plan.

6. Beans and Lentil – Beans, beans are good for your heart... Beans are low in fat (except for soybeans), calories, and sodium and are high in complex carbs and fiber. They are also an excellent source of protein. If you combine them with grains such as barley, brown rice, or oats, you will have all the amino acids necessary to make a complete protein. Eat your beans!

7. Fruit – Fruits are some of the healthiest and most natural foods you can eat. Fruit is packed with vitamins and minerals, and the great thing is that there are hundreds to choose from. I have heard a lot of people suggest that when you are trying to lose weight you should not eat fruit. That is bogus! I believe that fruit can actually help you with your weight control. Fruit is a good, convenient snack with a lot of health benefits. Fruits can reduce the risk of cardiovascular disease, lower blood pressure, lower cholesterol, reduce the risk of cancer, slow down the aging process, and reduce the chance of developing diabetes. Eat that fruit! Fruit does not take the place of your veggies. For the next 12 days, I want you to use a 1:3 ratio – one fruit for every three servings of veggies each day.

Day Sixteen

TRANSFORM YOUR BODY Today you will perform each exercise starting with 1 and finishing with 8. Remember, you will now perform each exercise for 30 sec, and rest for 15 sec. Perform 2 sets through all 8 exercises with 90 sec of rest in between sets.

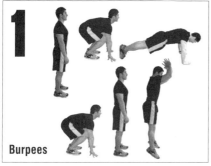

1 Burpees

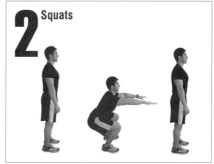

2 Squats

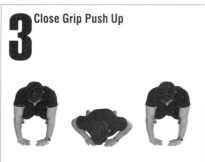

3 Close Grip Push Up

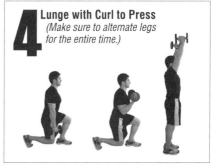

4 Lunge with Curl to Press
(Make sure to alternate legs for the entire time.)

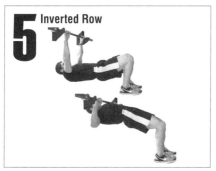

5 Inverted Row

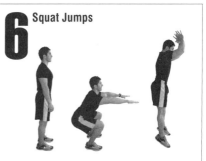

6 Squat Jumps

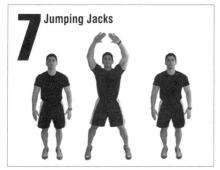

7 Jumping Jacks

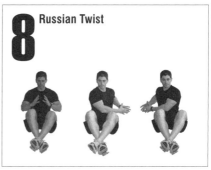

8 Russian Twist

Day Seventeen

THE SECRET
TO REAL WEIGHT LOSS SUCCESS

DO Expect Results

Today you will begin to expect results!

Preparation time is never wasted time. When you do what you need to do, then you should expect results. If you are following this game plan 100 percent, then you should expect to see the results you desire. The mind is a powerful weapon. If you don't believe in yourself, then why should anyone else believe in you? Starting today, I want you to develop a confidence that you are taking care of business, that you are back in the race, that you are going to finish it, and that you will not quit until you reach your final goal. Remember, the only one that can take you out of the game is yourself. Remember, the only one that can take you out of the race is you. Start expecting results, start expecting good things, and start expecting your life to take a turn in the right direction.

Right now, I want you to get out two pieces of paper. On the first sheet I want you to write down the positive results that you are expecting to see. On the other sheet I want you to write down an exact time that you would like to see those results by. Now take the two sheets and put them away for a later date.

Day
Seventeen

TRANSFORM YOUR EATING

The Hit List

These are the foods that today you will eliminate from your plan. I call this list the Hit List for a reason. These foods are detrimental to your success, and if you want to research it for yourself, go ahead. This is my official Hit List, and you need to stay away from these foods to be successful.

Coach JC's Hit List:

- Refined Sugar

- Artificial Sweeteners

- Trans-Fat Hydrogenated Oils (Fried Foods)

- White Flour Products

- Pork

- High Fructose Corn Syrup

- Most Fast Food

Starting today, your transformation is to eliminate these foods from your daily plan. If you eat them, it will be on your cheat day only.

Day Seventeen

TRANSFORM YOUR BODY Today you will perform each exercise starting with 1 and finishing with 8. Remember, you will now perform each exercise for 30 sec, and rest for 15 sec. Perform 2 sets through all 8 exercises with 90 sec of rest in between sets.

1 High Knees
(This is just like running in place. Get those knees up!)

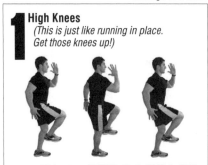

2 Rotational Push Ups
(Make sure to perform an even amount on each side. Alternate each rep.)

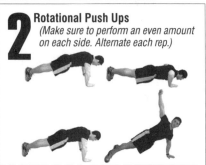

3 Split Squat
(Perform the movement on each leg for the designated time frame.)

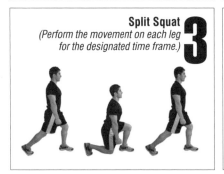

4 Body Builders

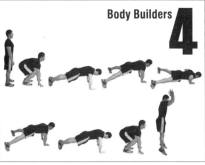

5 In and Outs
(Jump your feet out and in.)

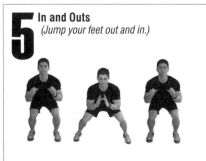

6 One Leg Push Ups

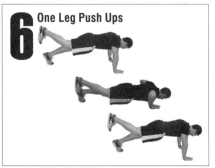

7 Crossing Jacks

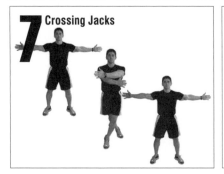

8 Split Squat Jumps
(Make sure to alternate legs each rep!)

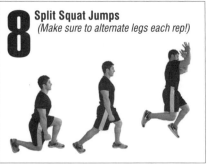

Day
Eighteen   THE SECRET
TO REAL WEIGHT LOSS SUCCESS

DISCOVER What You Sow You Shall Reap

What You Sow You Shall Reap.

You have probably heard this before, and I have found it to be very true in many different aspects of life. If you sow badly, you will reap badly; if you sow eating junk food you will reap the negative rewards of the junk food. You are what you eat, and you are what you think! That actually is very true. You have to start sowing well in what you eat, in your lifestyle, and in your fitness. As you start to sow, you will reap the benefits of eating well. As you sow exercise, you will see those pounds fall off or be put on, depending on your goal. Be excited about the body you are going to have, be excited about increasing your productivity in all that you, and be excited about being alive and having the opportunity to live life to the fullest. Don't be afraid to have some enthusiasm about what you are doing because this will become contagious. You will start to see other areas of your life improving. Remember, you have a fabulous future to look forward to and you should enjoy life today and every step along the way. Today, your transformation is to sow whatever it is that you want to reap. If you want to reap mediocre results then follow the game plan halfway, but if you want to experience ultimate fulfillment, then sow all that you can into this program for the next 10 days!

18

THE GAME PLAN

Day Eighteen

TRANSFORM YOUR EATING

Want To Go Out?

I don't know about you, but I like to eat out. There is nothing more fun to me then to take my fiancée out for a great romantic meal or to go out with friends for a fun night at a favorite restaurant. You may eat out often or you may eat out rarely. Regardless, I want to show you how you can make wise decisions while eating out. I don't care if you go to McDonald's or a fancy restaurant, you can always make a healthy, conscious decision.

Here are the keys to stay true to the plan while eating out:

1. Realize that the menu is just a suggestion list! If you do not see what you want on the menu, let the waiter know and create your own.

2. Follow the game plan! You must still follow the game plan, and if you do, you will be fine.

3. Always ask how foods are prepared or cooked. You want your items baked or grilled, and your veggies steamed and not soaked in butter. Ask for dressing on the side.

4. Many restaurants serve bread. If it is not a post-workout meal, just tell them "don't worry about bringing the bread."

5. If you know where you are going, do your homework ahead of time and figure out what you plan to have off of the menu. Almost all restaurants have an online menu, and many show nutritional facts for their items.

6. Enjoy Your Experience!!

Day Eighteen

TRANSFORM YOUR BODY Perform each exercise starting with 1 and finishing with 8. Perform each exercise for 30 sec, and now rest for only 10 sec. Perform 2 sets through all 8 exercises with 90 sec of rest in between sets.

1 Burpees with Push Up

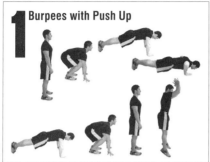

2 Plank
(Perform plank position for the designated time.)

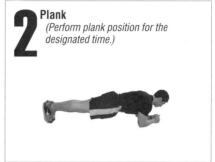

3 Pull Ups
(Beginners can perform jumping pull ups. Jump up to the top position and control the way down, then repeat.)

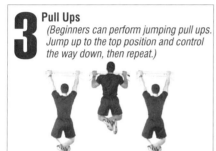

4 Push Up - Feet Elevated

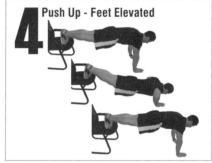

5 Squats

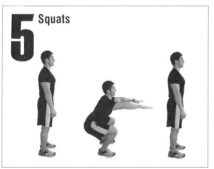

6 Side Lunge
(Perform each side for the designated time.)

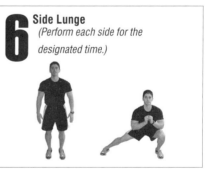

7 Mountain Climbers
(Continue to alternate legs for the entire time.)

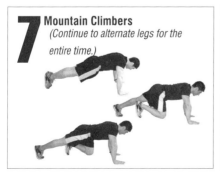

8 Long Striders
(Exaggerate the movement with big strides!)

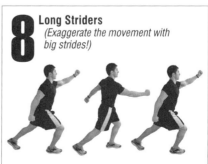

Day Nineteen

THE SECRET TO REAL WEIGHT LOSS SUCCESS

DO be a Control Freak

Starting today, you will be the one to control your future. Your future is up to you. Each decision that you make will determine where you are tomorrow. Your future is in your hands. You control your future, and you determine what happens tomorrow. This is your life; it is time for you to control the outcome of it. Starting today, you will not allow other people or situations to determine what happens in your life. No one made you fat! No one forced you to be who you are. You are in complete control of your life, and just one little decision can change your life forever. You will no longer allow your body to get so out of shape. Starting today, you will take control over the outcome. You have made the decision to be active and to exercise for these 27 days. You control your health. Be a control freak. Control your life, control your future, and control your destiny!

Your desire to be fit, to lose weight, and to conquer this area of your life must be strong; it must be strong enough to overcome mental laziness. Everyone wants the easy way out, but you do not any more. You are going to work for these results, and once they are achieved, they will work for you. They will continue to work for as long as you allow them to work for you. Today and every day from now on, you will make a conscious effort to make decisions that will better you and your future. You will become a control freak over who you are and who you want to be. Starting today, you will not allow anyone else to make decisions for you that will affect your life.

Day Nineteen

TRANSFORM YOUR EATING

Real Food or Supplements?

I am a fan of food supplementation. I believe it has benefits, but I want you to eat whole (real) foods first, whenever possible. Whole foods are richer in vitamins and minerals and provide enzymes, which guarantee that your body will process them, unlike most supplements. Supplements are very productive when used properly and implemented for the right reasons. With all the processed food out there today, it is difficult to obtain the nutrients that your body needs on a daily basis. People often use supplements to augment something that may be lacking in their plan or simply because of convenience. I believe it is best to mix whole foods and supplements. I want you to eat whole foods whenever possible and only use supplements for the times that it is more convenient for you. I recommend a few supplements simply because I don't believe people acquire enough nutrients in their daily plan. I recommended that most of my clients take a whole food multivitamin. Depending on the needs of the client, I may also recommend a protein powder, a greens drink, or fish oil. These are great supplements and I encourage you to do your research on these supplements.

Day Nineteen

TRANSFORM YOUR BODY Perform each exercise starting with 1 and finishing with 8. Perform each exercise for 30 sec, and now rest for only 10 sec. Perform 2 sets through all 8 exercises with 90 sec of rest in between sets.

1 Defensive Slide
(Perform 5 yards each side back and forth for the designated time.)

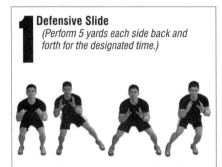

2 Curl Squat to Press

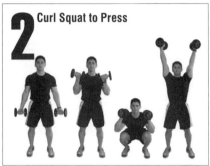

Body Builders 3

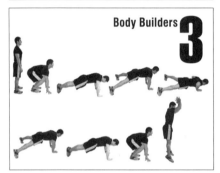

Inverted Row 4

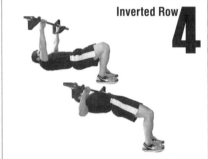

5 In and Outs
(Jump your feet out and in.)

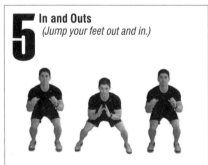

6 Step Up
(Alternate legs throughout the entire time - up, down, down, up.)

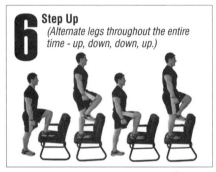

7 High Knees
(This is just like running in place. Get those knees up!)

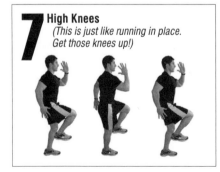

8 Push Up to Row

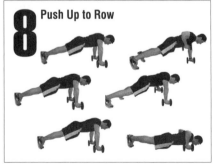

Day Twenty

THE SECRET TO REAL WEIGHT LOSS SUCCESS

DO Take Action

Today for your transformation you are going to take action! Just get moving! Start to make some forward progress. What have you been relaxed about in the past that has led you to put on weight and not live the life that you deserve? What can you do today to take action? Today, I want you to do something that you have not done before or have not done in many years. Maybe it is taking a walk, going for a run, riding a bike, taking a hike, or going for a swim. You get my point! I want you to do something active that you have not done in a long time. Today you will get out of your comfort zone by taking action. So many people say to me that they hate running. I ask them, "When was the last time you ran?" A lot of people then tell me that they haven't run since they were a kid, but they absolutely hated it. Oh course you hate it, because you never do it! It may be a little uncomfortable, but I don't care! Remember why you are doing this. Take action today! **NOT TOMORROW! TODAY!**

Day Twenty   TRANSFORM YOUR EATING

The Game Plan

You must keep this game plan with you at all times to be successful. Initially, I recommend that you keep it with you at all times so that you can reference it when needed. Once you master it, it will become a habit and a routine, and you will automatically apply the principles when you have to make choices. Your transformation for today is to make sure that from this day on, this game plan is always accessible to you. We have some clients who keep it in their purses or briefcases; others make copies, laminate the pages, and put them in a visible location, like the refrigerator or on their desk at work. You must find what works for you and make it work! This is your tool to be successful. Utilize it! Besides your Bible, this is the most important book to you!

Day Twenty

TRANSFORM YOUR BODY Today we are going to kick the intensity up a little more. Perform 3 sets through the workout instead of 2 like we have been for the last 3 weeks. Perform all 8 exercises, still starting with 1 and finishing with 8 with 90 sec of rest in between sets. Perform each exercise for 30 sec, and now rest for 15 sec.

1 High Pull / Squat to Press

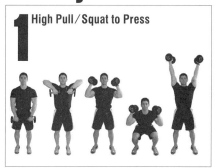

2 Dips

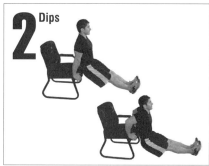

3 High Knees
(This is just like running in place. Get those knees up!)

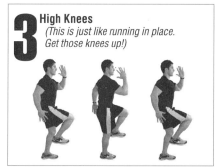

4 Lunge with Chop
(Make sure to perform each side for the designated time.)

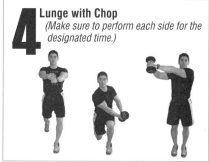

5 Plank
(Perform plank position for the designated time.)

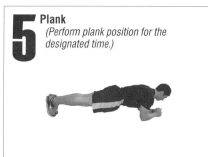

6 Crossing Jacks

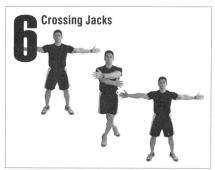

7 Pull Ups
(Beginners can perform jumping pull ups. Jump up to the top position and control the way down, then repeat.)

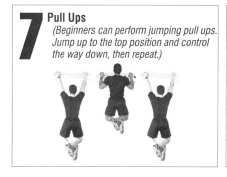

8 Close Grip Push Up

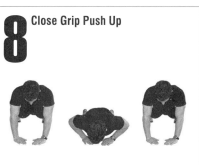

Day Twenty One

THE SECRET TO REAL WEIGHT LOSS SUCCESS

DO Become Agile

Today, your transformation is to become agile. How fast can you get from point A to point B? It is day 21, and by now, obstacles have probably occurred, times have been tough, and the road has been rocky, but I have already told you to expect this. The question is: what did you do when these inevitable circumstances happened? Did you fight through? Did you battle so that it did not slow your progress down? Hopefully you did! Obstacles will continue to appear, and for the rest of your life, you will have adversity when you try to do something good for yourself. Remember, when these obstacles come at you, you have to do whatever it takes to get through them. Nothing can stop you. I don't care if you have to go through, around, over, or under. Whatever you have to do, you must do it. You must make a conscious effort on a daily basis, and you must decide to fight though obstacles. When tough times come, go around them. Every day a situation will arise, so practice becoming more agile. Today, your transformation is to use daily circumstances to make you more agile so that when the large obstacles are thrown at you, they will not affect you. What do you need to do today to make sure that obstacles no longer slow you down?

Day Twenty One

TRANSFORM YOUR EATING

Go Organic?

What does organic mean? Organic farming excludes the use of chemicals and pesticides. Organic farms don't use synthetic fertilizers and don't feed growth hormones to the animals. Organic food is known to contain 50 percent more nutrients, minerals, and vitamins than produce that has been intensively farmed. Most poultry and cattle are force-fed antibiotics and hormones, and we digest those chemicals when we eat food that comes from those animals. These hormones, antibiotics, and pesticides in food have been linked to many diseases including cancer, obesity, Alzheimer's, and even some birth defects. I am not going to tell you that you should only buy organic foods. I am not even going to tell you that organic food is more nutritious or even safer than non-organic food, or that organic food is going to cure cancer because there is not enough evidence to prove that. I can tell you that with certain foods, it would be beneficial for you to buy organic. These include any fruits and vegetables that you do not peel before eating and all meats, poultry, and dairy products. You will still reach your weight-loss goals by eating non-organic foods, but remember, this is about more than just looking good. Today, I want you to try something organic to transform you and your family's overall health.

21

THE GAME PLAN

Day Twenty One

TRANSFORM YOUR BODY

R E C O V E R Y

Today you will be off from performing exercises so that your body can rest. Today you will stay active by doing something that you enjoy. I want for you to stay active doing something that you enjoy for at least 30 min!

TRY

- taking a walk

- playing at the park with your kids

- taking a bike ride

- playing a game

Have fun and get ready to kick it up tomorrow in your workout!

N O T E S :

_____

_____

_____

_____

_____

_____

_____

_____

_____

_____

Day Twenty Two

THE SECRET TO REAL WEIGHT LOSS SUCCESS

DETERMINE Your Priorities

22

THE GAME PLAN

Today, your transformation will be to address the priorities in your life. What are your priorities? A lot of people can define a priority, but few people prioritize their daily life and activities. A lot of times I talk with people, and they tell me their priorities. However, their actions often do not reflect what they tell me. Ultimately, your priorities are not expressed by what you believe and say they are, but by what your actions show on a daily basis. You may know in your heart that you want to lose weight and live a healthy lifestyle, but it is the action step that is slowing your progress down.

I want to give you five steps to make your priorities a priority:

1. Know what you want.

2. Write it out and make it clear.

3. Live it out and walk it out on a daily basis.

4. Associate yourself with people who have like priorities.

5. Give it a check up on a monthly basis to re-evaluate your list.

Today, your transformation is to prioritize your life using the five steps above. List your top seven priorities and begin to walk them out on a daily basis.

Day Twenty Two

TRANSFORM YOUR EATING

Are You Boring

Today for your transformation I want you to try something new! Today, I want you to try something you have never tried before. It amazes me how many of my clients have never tried some of best and most nutritious foods. It all depends on how you were brought up and where you were brought up. I had never eaten chicken fried steak until I was 28 years old and living in Oklahoma. People in Oklahoma thought I was crazy. Most people just don't eat chicken fried steak in Jersey; plus, my mom was a health nut! I am not telling you to eat chicken fried steak... it is definitely not on your plan! However, I do want you to try something new that is going to be beneficial for your body. Just pick something at the grocery store. You could try some collard, kale, fennel, okra, artichoke, arugula, or eggplant! Maybe you could try some zucchini, snap peas, alfalfa sprouts, Brussels sprouts, radishes, or some wheat grass. I know there are probably several vegetables or fruits that you have never tried. Today, get out of your eating comfort zone! You may even find something that you really enjoy!

Day Twenty Two

TRANSFORM YOUR BODY Perform each exercise starting with 1 and finishing with 8. Perform each exercise for 30 sec, and rest for 15 sec. Perform 3 sets through all 8 exercises with 90 sec of rest in between sets. Only six days left. Get after it!

1 Swings
(This is a continual movement using a weighted object of choice.)

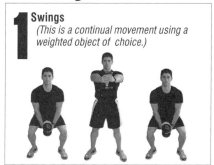

2 Curl Squat to Press

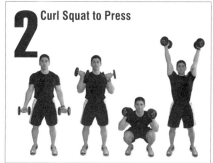

3 Side Plank
(Perform each side for the designated time.)

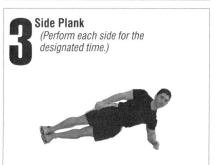

4 Inverted Row

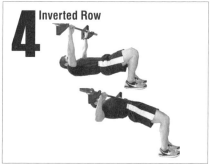

5 High Pull / Squat to Press

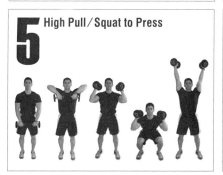

6 Pull Ups
(Beginners can perform jumping pull ups. Jump up to the top position and control the way down, then repeat.)

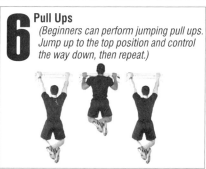

7 Russian Twists

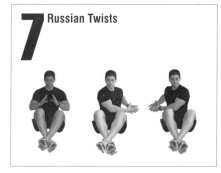

8 Squat Jumps

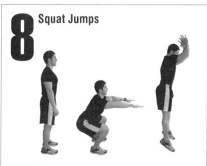

Day Twenty Three

THE SECRET TO REAL WEIGHT LOSS SUCCESS

DISCOVER Goal Setting

If you don't know what you want, you will never get it. If you don't know where you are going, you will never get there. Setting goals will help lead you to where you want to go in life. By knowing where you want to go, it enables you to concentrate your activities, actions, and efforts. I work with a lot of successful people, and they set goals. Look at successful athletes or even successful businessmen, they all set goals!

I am never surprised when I sit down with clients and ask them about their goals. They may say that they want to play in the NBA, lose weight, put on 25 pounds of muscle, or just be healthy. A lot of people have defined their ultimate long-term goal, which is a great first step. However, when I ask them what they are doing to reach that goal, very few people have the steps, the short-term goals, mapped out. Your short-term goals are going to lead to that ultimate goal. What do you need to do on a daily, weekly, and monthly basis to get to your ultimate goal? Today for your transformation, you will complete a goal worksheet. First, you will write down your ultimate goal. For example, maybe you want to lose 80 pounds. Next, you are going to map out short-term goals to lead you to that 80-pound weight loss. Plan out what are you going to do on a daily basis, on a weekly basis, and maybe even on an annual basis until you reach that 80-pound weight-loss goal. Here is a hint: you already have the answer in your hands; it is called the game plan! Get after it!

Day Twenty Three

TRANSFORM YOUR EATING

Healthy Snacking!

What can I eat for my snacks? What can I pack on the road when I am traveling? I get these questions all of the time. Here are a few great options: fruit, raw veggies, hardboiled eggs, mixed nuts, and seeds. Eating healthy snacks on the road comes down to planning and preparing in advance, just like we talked about on day nine. It is easier to have these snacks with you, then to have to figure out where to stop and what to eat. Fortunately, if you need to stop, a lot fast food and convenience stores are now carrying healthy options for snacks. You just need to have some knowledge on what to purchase. Watch out for some of the protein or meal replacement bars out there; just because they are marketed as being healthy does not mean that they are. A lot of these bars are very high in calories and fat, and most of these bars are packed with high fructose corn syrup and hydrogenated oils. These cheap, unhealthy ingredients are used by manufactures to add flavor to the bars. As you already know, both of them are on our "Hit List" from day 17.

Some other healthy snacks are almond butter, cashew butter, peanut butter, fat-free cottage cheese, fat-free yogurt, dried fruit, and hummus. Be creative and enjoy your snacks; just make sure your snacks are compliant with the game plan.

Day Twenty Three

TRANSFORM YOUR BODY Perform each exercise starting with 1 and finishing with 8. Perform each exercise for 30 sec, and rest for 15 sec. Perform 3 sets through all 8 exercises with 90 sec of rest in between sets. How bad do you want it?

Body Builders **1**

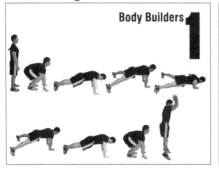

Negative Push Ups **2**
(Take 5 seconds on the way down.)

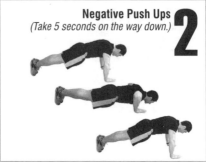

3 Defensive Slide
(Perform 5 yards each side back and forth for the designated time.)

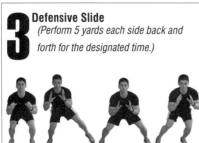

4 Lunge with Curl to Press
(Make sure to alternate legs for the entire time.)

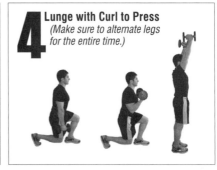

5 High Knees
(This is just like running in place. Get those knees up!)

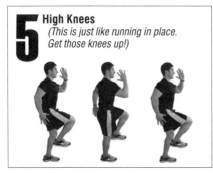

6 Push Up - Feet Elevated

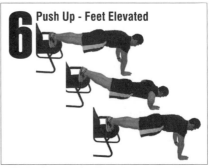

7 Mountain Climbers
(Continue to alternate legs for the entire time.)

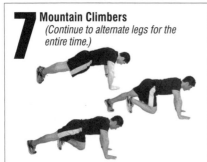

8 Step Up
(Alternate legs throughout the entire time - up, down, down, up.)

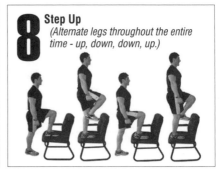

Day Twenty Four

THE SECRET TO REAL WEIGHT LOSS SUCCESS

DECIDE To Speak It

Today, you will begin to speak those things that you desire and want to accomplish. I want you to speak with confidence and a positive attitude and believe, without a doubt, that the things you are working at will work out. If you want to lose 20 pounds, then keep telling yourself, "I am going to lose these 20 pounds!" Remember, this will subconsciously make you find ways to lose those 20 pounds. On the other hand, don't ever allow yourself to say, "I'll never lose these 20 pounds." Starting today, you have to believe that what you speak is powerful and is a huge component in accomplishing your goal. Remember, some people do not want to see you succeed, and they doubt that you can do this. You will never really experience true success in your life until you master your speaking. By now, you probably know that I am big on action, but I have found that combining the power of speaking with action is incredible! You are not only speaking it, but you are putting action behind it. This is what the game plan is all about, and this is what you have been doing for the last 23 days. It is a powerful combination! So, let me speak into your life again and tell you I believe in you and I believe that you will accomplish your goal. I don't care if you want to lose 10 pounds or 250 pounds, I believe you can do it and I believe you will not quit until you get there. I have faith in you. Your transformation is to speak your goal out loud five times throughout the day. Speak it to achieve it!

Day Twenty Four

TRANSFORM YOUR EATING

Are You Counting Calories?

I know by now that at least a few of you count your calories. Like I told you in the beginning, you do not need to count calories on this program to be successful. Counting calories to me is not much fun, but I have some clients who are accountants and they beg to differ. I understand that some of you may want to count your calories, and I always get a lot of emails in regards to this, so I have provided some information here. If you want to count your calories, here is a simple formula to figure out how many calories you need each day.

IF WEIGHT LOSS IS YOUR GOAL

Sedentary (minimal exercise)	Bodyweight Pounds x 10-12
Moderately Active (3-4 times/wk)	Bodyweight Pounds x 12-14
Very Active (5-7 times/wk)	Bodyweight Pounds x 14-16

If you do not want to count your calories, then just continue to follow the game plan. Today, I want you to revisit each of the past days and make sure you are still following the plan to a T. If there is an area that you need to reevaluate, DO IT NOW!

Day Twenty Four

24

THE GAME PLAN

1 Forward Lunge
(Alternate legs like you are walking. Perform an even amount on each leg.)

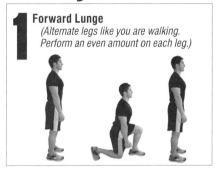

2 Squat to Press

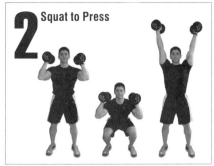

3 Reverse Lunge
(Make sure to alternate legs each rep!)

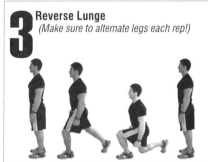

4 Burpees

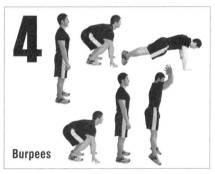

5 Rotational Push Up

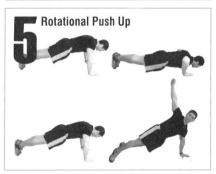

6 Pull Up

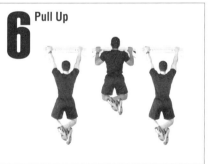

7 Plank
(Perform plank position for the designated time.)

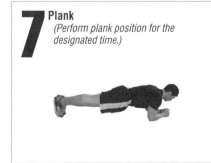

8 Jumping Jacks

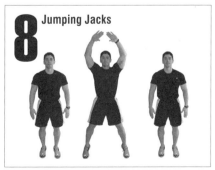

Day Twenty Five

THE SECRET TO REAL WEIGHT LOSS SUCCESS

DO Realize That It is a Choice

It is a choice, and it is your decision! How badly do you really want it? How badly do you really want to be in shape? How badly do you really want to lose weight? How badly do you really want to live a fulfilled life? Well, I have great news for you. Go and live that great, fulfilled life! Go and get into the best shape of your life! Go and lose that weight! Now is your time. Today, I want you to make a decision that you are not going to live another day on cruise control. Make a decision that you are not going to allow your life to become stagnant. Starting today, I want you to have passion about who you are and what you are doing. You will no longer allow others to make decisions for you! You will no longer allow other people to choose your future! You may not have the perfect body, you may not have the perfect job, you may not live in the perfect environment, but remember, you can choose to change any of that, today! You are choosing to take control of your life. You are choosing to take your life back! Today, you are choosing to take control of your health by taking control of your thinking. You choose your future, you choose what your body looks like, you choose how much money you make, and you choose what religion you practice. It's your choice! You are in control, and starting today, I want you to transform your life by making wise choices.

Day Twenty Five

TRANSFORM YOUR EATING

Are You Compliant?

Your success depends on you! Remember, this game plan will not fail you. The only way you will not see results is if you fail the game plan. Your success depends on if you are being compliant with the plan. Are you taking care of business? Are you doing what you need to be doing? Are you being adherent to the plan and sticking to it 100%? You have all the tools that you need to succeed, so I want to ask you a quick question: are you giving it 100% every day? Well, let's find out! For your transformation today you will measure your compliance. Here is what I want for you to do. Take out a piece of paper and write down the numbers 1 through 24 on the left side of the paper. Then go back to day one and honestly answer the question, "Have I followed the plan 100% for today?" Next to the number on your paper, you will either put a "yes" or a "no." Now you will do this for each day up to this point. Remember, once you complete a day, you must continue to apply that day's key every day for the entire 27 days. It is as simple as that. Yes or no, either you have been following it 100% or you have not. Make the necessary adjustments so that you are 100% compliant and are adhering to the game plan. If you are, you can experience what hundreds of other people are already experiencing: true happiness and success!

Day Twenty Five

TRANSFORM YOUR BODY Perform each exercise starting with 1 and finishing with 8. Perform each exercise for 30 sec, and rest for 10 sec. Perform 3 sets through all 8 exercises with 90 sec of rest in between sets. Only 3 days left. Finish Strong!

1 Burpees with Push Up

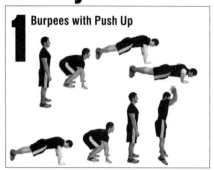

2 Side Plank
(Perform each side for the designated time.)

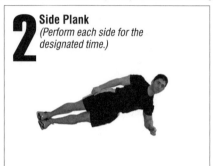

3 Lunge with Curl to Press
(Make sure to alternate legs for the entire time.)

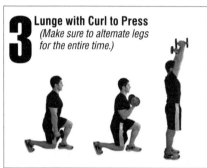

4 Russian Twist

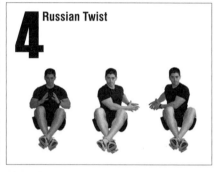

5 High Knees
(This is just like running in place. Get those knees up!)

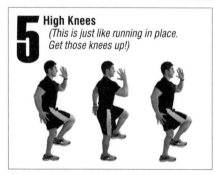

6 Plank
(Perform plank position for the designated time.)

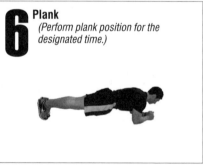

7 Inverted Row

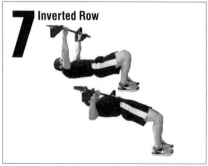

8 Defensive Slide
(Perform 5 yards each side back and forth for the designated time.)

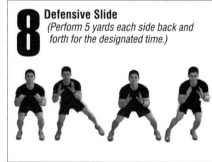

Day Twenty Six

THE SECRET TO REAL WEIGHT LOSS SUCCESS

DO Believe In Yourself

You have been made with a purpose, and you can do this! You have to be optimistic about yourself, you have to believe in your dreams, and you have to believe that you are going to achieve those things. You have to believe that you are going to lose that desired weight now because you have changed your thinking and have been implementing the game plan. Believe that now is your time and believe that this is the body that you deserve. Starting today, your transformation is to believe in yourself and portray a confidence of belief. Today, your transformation has three steps:

1. Watch your body language. I don't care what situation you are in; you must have nothing but positive body language. This will help you get in the right mindset and also project confidence to the people around you.

2. Watch your thinking. I don't care what the problem is; don't get off the plan. Don't get angry; instead, just handle it and move on. Avoid thinking negatively. Today, you must start to look at problems as potential solutions and allow them to build your self-confidence. Look for a solution to the problem and allow it to improve your life. What can you learn from it?

3. Avoid negative people. Avoid anyone who tries to take you down or criticize you. Some of these people may think that they are helping you or that they are trying to prevent you from failing. Do not listen to them! You are following your goals, and you will be successful. Follow your game plan!

Day Twenty Six

TRANSFORM YOUR EATING

Fiber it up!

Fiber is important to your success during this 27-day transformation.

It has been proven that getting enough fiber in the diet can lower the risk of certain health conditions like heart disease, cancer, diabetes, gallstones, and kidney stones. Besides preventing certain diseases, fiber offers some other great health benefits. It can help relieve constipation and hemorrhoids and can assist in keeping your weight under control.

Your transformation today is to start incorporating more fiber into you daily plan. There are two types of fiber, and you want to make sure you are getting a combination of both.

- **Insoluble fiber** – can be found in nuts, wheat bran, whole grains, and most vegetables.

- **Soluble fiber** – can be found in citrus fruit (oranges and lemons), apples, beans, oats, and barley grain.

However, as with a lot of things in life, too much of a good thing can become a bad thing. The amount of fiber you should get throughout the day depends on your weight, but here is a good guideline to start with since most of us lack fiber in our daily eating habits.

Adults over 50 years of age: 21g for women or 30g for men

Adults under 50 years of age: 25g for women or 38g for men

Day Twenty Six

TRANSFORM YOUR BODY Perform each exercise starting with 1 and finishing with 8. Perform each exercise for 30 sec, and rest for 10 sec. Perform 3 sets through all 8 exercises with 90 sec of rest in between sets. Go as hard as you can go! Only 2 days left!

Step Up **1**
(Alternate legs through out the entire time - up, down, down, up.)

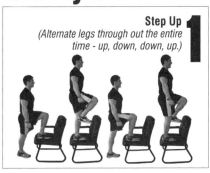

Body Builders **2**

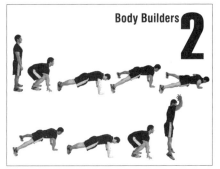

3 Push Ups

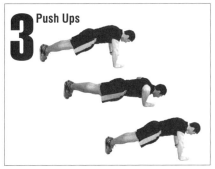

4 Mountain Climbers
(Continue to alternate legs for the entire time.)

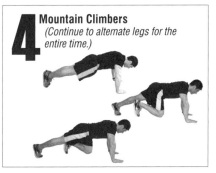

5 In and Outs
(Jump your feet out and in.)

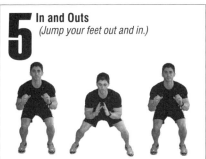

6 Swings
(This is a continual movement using a weighted object of choice.)

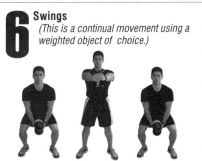

7 Pull Ups
(Beginners can perform jumping pull ups. Jump up to the top position and control the way down, then repeat.)

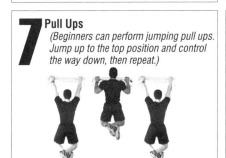

8 Split Squat Jumps
(Make sure to alternate legs each rep!)

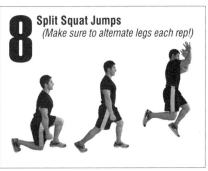

Day Twenty Seven

THE SECRET TO REAL WEIGHT LOSS SUCCESS

DO Just Do It

Now is your time! You know that the last 27 days were not easy, but if you have been following the game plan, your life should be drastically different. How badly do you really want this? I want you to really think about this: in just 27 days your life has changed. The way you think, look, and feel is different because you decided to just do it! My challenge for you now is, can you continue to give it everything that you have? Can you continue to do it like there is no tomorrow? Is your life worth it? Actions speak louder than words, so show me what you've got! Your transformation for today is to not stop! Keep going strong until you reach your ultimate goal. This 27-day plan was just the beginning, and now, you have developed a habit, so why not continue what you are doing? For 27 days you did it! Now, just keep doing it!!!

Go to **www.CaochJC.com**

and get your next 27 days of

Your 27 Day Body Transformation Gameplan!

Day Twenty Seven

TRANSFORM YOUR EATING

Watch How You Cook

Your transformation today is to master your cooking. A lot of people do not realize that calories can add up from the way they are preparing their food. Starting today, I want you to make a few changes if you have not already. Try to always grill, bake, or broil your meats, poultry, and fish. Make wise decisions on your choice of sauces and marinades when cooking these foods. Your best bet is to use some seasonings. A lot of great tasting, low-calorie seasonings are out there. When it comes to vegetables, I want you to steam or stir-fry them. If you cook with lard, butter, palm oil, or coconut oil, stop! Starting today, you will cook with unsaturated vegetable oils, such as corn, olive, canola, safflower, sesame, soybean, sunflower, or peanut. Your best bet is to use a stick-free pan with very little or no oil; fat-free cooking spray is the best way to go.

Day Twenty Seven

TRANSFORM YOUR BODY Perform each exercise starting with 1 and finishing with 8. Perform each exercise for 30 sec. and rest for 10 sec. Perform 3 sets through all 8 exercises with 90 sec of rest in between sets. Finish Strong! One more workout and you did it!

1 Rotational Push Ups
(Make sure to perform an even amount on each side. Alternate each rep.)

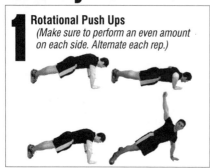

2 Squat Jumps

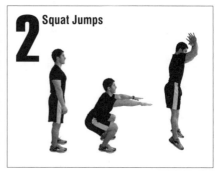

3 Inverted Row

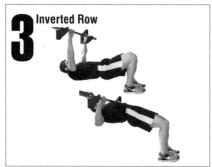

4 High Knees
(This is just like running in place. Get those knees up!)

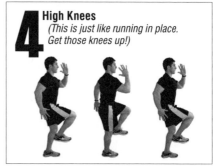

5 High Pull / Squat to Press

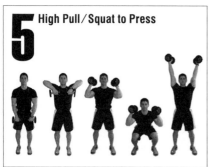

6 Burpees

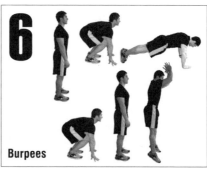

7 Lunge with Curl to Press
(Make sure to alternate legs for the entire time.)

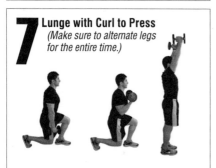

8 Plank
(Perform plank position for the designated time.)

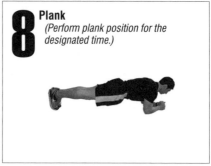

THE CHARGE

Congratulations! You have completed your 27-Day Transformation. I want to first say that I am proud of you! I know you feel better and look better. This is not the end but only the beginning. By now you should be in a routine, and you have made the lifestyle changes to take your life to the next level. I want to challenge you to continue. You have changed your life forever! You are not a part of the norm any more! Keep going strong!

I want to warn you that most of the people who are around you are not like you any longer. You have made a decision to be your best while they may still be satisfied with mediocrity. They may be satisfied with just going through the motions while you, from now on, will always want more out of life.

You have stepped out of your comfort zone and have lived a little on the edge so that you could experience more and see your dreams become a reality. You took a risk! The people around you may not understand why you don't want to be satisfied and content any longer. You chose to no longer just live the safe way but rather, take the risks to achieve great things and be successful. People will still try to talk you out of what you are doing and will tell you that you are crazy. Do you know why? It is because they are scared of success and they really want what you have. They are scared to take the risk that you have taken for the last 27 days because they do not possess the same mindset that you do. They will tell you that there is always tomorrow and that there is time. There is tomorrow, but time moves quickly, so don't wait until you are ten years older to look back with regret. You will still face obstacles and tough times, but now it will no longer slow you down because you want this so badly that you are willing to never quit. This book was created to get you back in the right direction, to give you that kick-start that you needed.

I knew what you needed and I gave it to you. Now I am here to support you, and trust me, you can do it! When I started my Bootcamp Tulsa program, people told me that I couldn't do it and that it wouldn't work. However, we now have five locations with multiple times available, and we are helping over 250 women a week in Tulsa to transform their bodies and their lives.

Do you know why? Because I never quit and I will never quit! I have too many people counting on me and now you do also. This is about you. This is your life, and you need to be able to look back with no regret. You need to be able to look in the mirror and know that you are living the life that you deserve.

Now show everyone what you've got! Start your next 27 days holding nothing back.

Don't forget to send me your testimonials and keep me posted on your progress. You are now a part of the family... Here's to a Healthier, Happier, and more Successful you!

Make sure to visit

www.CoachJC.com

to get all of your body transformation tools!

CONGRATULATIONS!

You did it! You completed your 27-day game plan so that you can have anything you want anytime that you want it in business and in life.

The principles that you have just read are simple, and they work if you just work them. Once you transform your thinking, you will be able to have that thing or things that you so badly desire.

THE CHOICE IS YOURS, MY FRIEND!

Remember, success is not some big event that just happens. It comes down to you executing your daily action steps and exercising the law of compound in your life. No one else can do it for you. Time can work for you or against you! What's your choice? How badly do you want this success?

I believe in you and know that you desperately want it. Listen to me, don't get overwhelmed, just follow the game plan and execute that one simple, disciplined thing every day that will get you to the promise land!

SO, WHERE DO YOU GO FROM HERE?

You go back to page one of this book and you go through every day again to assure that you are executing the game plan. Remember, retention without implementation is useless... What are you going to do with it?

KEEP IT SIMPLE! HAVE FUN! AND REMEMBER,
YOUR LIFE IS WHAT YOU MAKE IT!

Coach JC,

DO YOU NEED TO LOSE WEIGHT & GET FIT?

GET YOUR **27- DAY BODY TRANSFORMATION GAME PLAN** NOW!

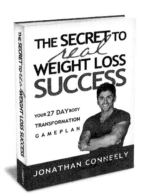

You Will Discover The Secret To:

- **Achieve The Body** You Have Always Desired
- **Look And Feel Great** About Yourself Again
- **Be Healthier** And Live A More Abundant Life

GET YOUR COPY TODAY!

Ask about discounts for schools or organizations ordering large quantities; please call **1 800-382-1506**

W W W . C O A C H J C . C O M

 facebook.com/Jonathan.Conneely   @Coach_JC

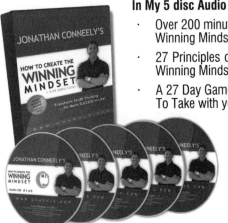

DO YOU WANT TO ACHIEVE MORE

IN BUSINESS AND IN LIFE?

GET **YOUR 27 DAY BUSINESS & LIFE GAME PLAN** NOW!

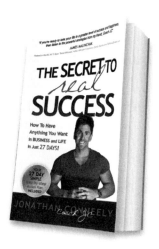

GET
YOUR
COPY
TODAY!

·   Discover how to have anything you want anytime you want!

·   Create the life you were born to live!

·   Be more and achieve more starting today!

WWW.COACHJC.COM

facebook.com/Jonathan.Conneely   @Coach_JC

TITLE	COPIES	PRICE	TOTAL
The Secret to Real Success		$14.99	
Shipping/Handling		$3.00 For 1-2 Books	
Make checks or money orders payable to: JJC Enterprises 8177 S Harvard Ave., Suite 420, Tulsa OK 74137		**TOTAL**	

REQUEST COACH JC FOR YOUR NEXT EVENT

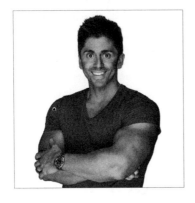

For over 12 years now Coach JC has been motivating individuals and organizations to Live more and Achieve More.

It's Time for YOU To Take It To The NEXT LEVEL!

I WOULD LOVE TO HEAR FROM YOU!

I know this book has changed your life! I would love to hear from you. Please write to me as I would love to hear how it has touched your life.

Contact me! Send letters to:
Coach JC
JJC Enterprises
8177 S Harvard Ave.
Suite 420
Tulsa, OK 74137

email or call us:
1 800-382-1506
email: jc@coachjc.com
website: www.CoachJC.com

Scan with a smartphone to connect with me on Facebook or Twitter

COACH JC , YOUR LIFE SUCCESS COACH

coaches people on a daily basis on how to experience Optimal Wellness and True Success in their life! As a Lifestyle, Fitness and Strength Coach, Coach JC's No Nonsense, No Excuse approach has been transforming lives for over 12 years now.

As an established Author, Speaker, and Coach he is regarded as one of the top Coaches in the entire country. He has been assisting individuals from all walks of life to "Take it to the next level!" Coach JC motivates people to take control of their life. Coach JC has a passion for helping people live the life they were born to live.

He is the Founder and President of JJC Enterprises, Life Coaching. He is the Founder of the well-recognized Sports Performance Company, Dynamic Sports Development, and the Founder of Bootcamp Tulsa, Tulsa's first ever, outdoor fitness program. Bootcamp Tulsa has been named one of the country's Top 10 Outdoor Fitness Bootcamps.

In addition, Coach JC is the Director of Strength and Conditioning at an NCAA Division I institution and the Creator of The Secret To REAL Weight Loss Success...FOR CHRISTIANS. Coach JC's coaching philosophy remains consistent in that he is dedicated to providing the tools necessary to empower individuals to create Ultimate Lifestyle Changes.

Coach JC's qualifications include a Bachelors of Science degree, a Life Coach certification, multiple coaching, sports performance and fitness certifications, with none more valuable than his 12 years in the trenches. He is the author of The Secret To Real Weight Loss Success, Your 27 Day Body Transformation Game plan, co-author of the well recognized personal development book, The Code, as well as countless articles. He has also been a consultant to professional athletes, corporations, pageant contestants, businessmen, entrepreneurs, pastors, and others just like you.

Coach JC also inspires and coaches young entrepreneurs on how to follow their dreams and turn their passions into profits! He shows people how they can profit doing what they love to do, run their businesses with integrity, and make money at the same time!

GET MORE SUCCESS TOOLS AT

www.CoachJC.com